the fast diet

'The most popular diet this century'
Daily Telegraph

'The diet that has made even the sceptics sit up and listen'
Sainsbury's Magazine

'Dieting has never been so delicious'
Daily Mail

'Fasting two days in seven isn't so hard, unlike the diets
that need steely resolve 24/7'
Express

'The only diet you'll ever need'
Mail on Sunday

---

the fast diet

DR MICHAEL MOSLEY
& MIMI SPENCER

Photographs by Romas Foord

Nutritional advice and food styling by Annie Hudson

Published in 2014 by Short Books
Unit 316, ScreenWorks, 22 Highbury Grove,
London, N5 2ER

10 9 8 7

A CIP catalogue record for this book
is available from the British Library.

ISBN 978-1-78072-237-5

Printed in Great Britain by CPI Group (UK) Ltd. Croydon, CR0 4YY

For my wife Clare and children Alex, Jack, Daniel and Kate – who make living longer worthwhile. *MM*

———————————

For Ned, Lily May and Paul – my Brighton rock. And for my parents, who have always known that food is love. *MS*

CONTENTS

Foreword

On my first day as a medical student at the Royal Free Hospital School of Medicine, part of the University of London, I sat down with a hundred others in a huge lecture theatre to be greeted by the Dean. He talked for over an hour about how lucky we were to be there, our potentially glorious future and the importance of being kind to patients.

There are, however, two things he said that I still remember very clearly. The first was that, based on previous experience, four of us in that room would marry. He was right; I met my future wife that day.

The other thing he said which really struck me was that while we would learn an enormous amount over the first five years of our training, within ten years of graduating much of what we had learnt would be out of date.

Medicine and nutrition are disciplines in which the 'truth' is constantly changing. New studies come along, sometimes reinforcing and sometimes undermining established wisdom. Unless you keep up with the latest research you are doomed to cling to outdated ideas.

It has been two years since we wrote the first edition of

The Fast Diet and over that time a great deal has changed, so we decided it was time to update the book.

A number of new studies on intermittent fasting have been published and I wanted to include them. There are also important health areas which we didn't feel ready to include in the original book, but which we have been frequently asked about, including research into the effects of intermittent fasting on inflammatory diseases such as asthma, eczema and psoriasis.

We have included an enlarged section on exercise, as it is clear that combining exercise with intermittent fasting is likely to lead to greater improvements. There is also an interesting new study that has looked at the effects of combining intermittent fasting with a novel form of exercise, High Intensity Training.

Then there's the all-important question of what you should eat on your fasting days. Mimi has created a whole new range of tasty and satisfying recipes, together with plenty of useful tips on how to shop and cook to best suit your Fast Days.

She has also put together a new section looking at motivation, based in part on what those who have tried the diet have told us.

The original book has sold in over 42 countries, making intermittent fasting into a truly international phenomenon. Although there are many different forms of intermittent fasting (and we discuss most of them in this book), 5:2, a term which I used to describe my particular form (cutting your calories to a quarter for two days a week) is the one that people seem to find easiest to do and which has become the most firmly embedded in the national psyche.

We're told that 5:2 has been embraced by celebrities like Beyoncé and Benedict Cumberbatch; it has become the diet of choice for government ministers, for the Chancellor of the Exchequer and the former Governor of the Bank of England; we have had messages of thanks from doctors, surgeons, parish priests, business leaders, sports teachers, school heads, politicians and a Nobel prize winner.

We set up a website (thefastdiet.co.uk) which is thriving and whose members support others who are thinking of trying intermittent fasting with helpful advice and tips. I have learnt a great deal from their experiences and questions.

The website contains thousands of success stories. These are a small sample:

> 'I heard the author on a radio show and he made so much sense I tried the diet. I have never stayed on a diet before. I lost 40lb in a few months. It is six months later and the weight is still gone.'

> 'I've now lost about 19lb in five weeks, my body fat is down from 37% to 33% and

I can take my jeans off without undoing them and am happy to do so if anyone will watch!'

'My body shape has changed beyond recognition. My muffin top has gone and I have gained a waist instead! I have been doing this for 21 weeks and have lost 19lb, but also 3" off my waist, 3" off my hips, 2" off each thigh. My psoriasis has gone too. I am 42… and looking the best I have for 20 years.'

Nothing works for everyone and some people have struggled to make it work for them. We include an updated 'troubleshooting' Q&A section to offer some helpful pointers to maximise your chances of success.

So why does it work?

In the first half of this book I delve into the science behind intermittent fasting. But one of the main reasons I think that the Fast Diet has been so successful is psychological. When you are on the 5:2 diet you aren't on a constant treadmill, dieting all the time.

I certainly find it easier to resist the temptation to eat a bar of chocolate by saying to myself, 'I will have it tomorrow.' Then tomorrow comes and maybe I eat it. But sometimes I don't.

Intermittent fasting also teaches you better ways of eating. If you follow our recipes and satisfy your hunger on fasting days by eating vegetables and good protein, then over time you'll discover that when you get hungry you are more likely to crave the healthy stuff. As someone recently wrote to me: 'You don't get cravings, you don't spend money on special foods or programs. I lost more than 25lb and my husband lost more than 35lb. It was easy to do and we have maintained the weight loss, even over the holidays. I wish I had discovered this method 30 years ago.'

The question I get asked most often is, not surprisingly, 'Are you still doing it?' The answer is, 'yes and no'. Back in the summer of 2012 I lost nearly 20lb (8kg), most of it fat, on the 5:2 diet. I also saw some spectacular improvements in things like my fasting glucose levels.

I didn't, however, want to go on losing weight, so I switched to doing mainly 6:1 (cutting my calories just one day a week). That, along with a regime of Fast Exercise (which I describe on pages 82-89) has kept my weight stable for the last two years. Stable, that is, apart from Christmas and the occasional lapse.

I can honestly say I am in far better shape than I was two years ago and I'm delighted so many other people can say the same.

Like me, Mimi is following a 6:1 protocol, and the

weight she lost in the first six months of the Fast Diet (7kg) has stayed off for good. If there's a blow-out for birthdays or holidays, she turns the dial back up to 5:2 and soon gets back on track. One of her greatest joys is her father's progress on the Fast Diet: after decades of being overweight, he lost over four stone in a single year – an astounding, life-changing achievement. As he says, 'It's not like dieting at all; these days, I barely notice I'm doing it. Since New Year's Day, I can only remember being hungry once.'

We both hope you enjoy this updated book and look forward to hearing more from you.

Michael Mosley, December 2014

FASTING: A BIT OF BACKGROUND...

Over the last few decades, food fads have come and gone, but the standard medical advice on what constitutes a healthy lifestyle has stayed much the same: eat low-fat foods, exercise more... and never, ever skip meals. Over that same period, levels of obesity have soared. Now many of those old certainties are being questioned.

When we first read about the benefits of intermittent fasting, we, like many, were sceptical. Fasting seemed drastic, difficult – and we both knew that dieting, of any description, is generally doomed to fail. But now that we've looked at it in depth and tried it ourselves, we are convinced of its remarkable potential. As one of the medical experts interviewed for this book puts it: 'There is nothing else you can do to your body that is as powerful as fasting.'

An ancient idea, a modern method

Fasting is nothing new. As we'll discover in the next chapter, your body is designed to fast. We evolved at a time when food was scarce; we are the product of millennia of feast and famine. The reason we respond so well to intermittent fasting is that it mimics, far more accurately than three meals a day, the environment in which modern humans were shaped.

Fasting, of course, remains an article of faith for many. The fasts of Lent, Yom Kippur and Ramadan are just some of the better-known examples. Greek Orthodox Christians are encouraged to fast for 180 days of the year (according to Saint Nikolai of Zicha, 'Gluttony makes a man gloomy and fearful, but fasting makes him joyful and courageous'), while Buddhist monks fast on the new moon and full moon of each lunar month.

Many more of us, however, seem to be eating most of the time. We're rarely ever hungry. But we are dissatisfied. With our weight, our bodies, our health.

Intermittent fasting can put us back in touch with our human selves. It is a route not only to weight loss, but also to long-term health and wellbeing. Scientists are only just beginning to discover and prove how powerful a tool it can be.

A review article recently published in the scientific journal, *Cell Metabolism*,[1] which looked at some of the most recent human and animal studies, makes the point that 'Fasting has been practised for millennia, but, only recently, studies have shed light on its role in adaptive cellular responses that reduce oxidative damage and inflammation, optimise energy metabolism, and bolster cellular protection.'

In other words, we now know that fasting reduces many of the things that promote ageing ('oxidative damage and inflammation') while increasing the body's ability to protect and repair itself ('cellular protection').

The article concludes that fasting 'helps reduce obesity, hypertension, asthma, and rheumatoid arthritis. Thus, fasting has the potential to delay ageing and help prevent and treat diseases.'

This book is a product of cutting-edge scientific research and its impact on our current thinking about weight loss, disease resistance and longevity. But it is also the result of our personal experience. Both are relevant here – the lab and the lifestyle – so we investigate intermittent fasting from two complementary perspectives. First, Michael, who used his body and medical training to test its potential, explains the scientific foundations of intermittent fasting and the 5:2 diet – something he brought to the world's attention back in the summer of 2012.

Then Mimi offers a practical guide on how to do it safely, effectively and in a sustainable way, a way that will fit easily into your normal, everyday life. She looks in detail at how fasting feels, what you can expect from day to day, what to eat and when to eat – and provides a host of tips and strategies to help you gain the greatest benefit from the diet's simple precepts.

As you'll see below, the Fast Diet has changed both of our lives. We hope it will do the same for you.

Michael's motivation: a male perspective

I am a 57-year-old male and before I embarked on my exploration of intermittent fasting I was mildly over-weight: at 5'11", I weighed around 85kg (13 stone 6lb) and had a Body Mass Index (BMI) of 26. Until my mid-30s, I had been slim, but like many people I then gradually put on weight, around 0.5kg a year. This doesn't sound much, but over a couple of decades it pushed me up and up. Slowly I realised that I was starting to resemble my father, a man who struggled with his weight all his life and died in his early 70s of complications associated with diabetes. At his funeral many of his friends commented on how like him I had become.

I was fortunate enough, while making a documentary for the BBC, to have an MRI scan done. This revealed that I am a TOFI, Thin on the Outside and Fat Inside. Fat on the inside – visceral fat – is the most dangerous sort of fat because it wraps itself around your internal organs and puts you at risk of heart disease and diabetes. I later had blood tests that showed I was heading towards diabetes, with a cholesterol score that was also way too high. Clearly I was going to have to do something about this. I tried following standard advice. Except it made little difference. My weight and blood profile remained stuck in the 'danger ahead' zone.

I had never tried dieting before because I'd never found a diet that I thought would work. I watched my father try every form of diet, from Scarsdale through Atkins, from the Cambridge Diet to the Drinking Man's Diet. He lost weight on each one of them, and then within a few months put it all back on, and more.

Then, at the beginning of 2012, I was approached by Aidan Laverty, editor of the BBC science series *Horizon*, who asked if I would like to put myself forward as a guinea pig to explore the science behind life extension. I wasn't sure what we would find, but, along with producer Kate Dart and researcher Roshan Samarasinghe, we quickly focused on calorie restriction and fasting as a fruitful area to explore.

Calorie restriction is pretty brutal; it involves eating an awful lot less than a normal person would expect to eat, and doing so every day of your – hopefully – long life. The reason people put themselves through this is that it is the only intervention that has been shown to extend lifespan, at least in animals. There are around 50,000 CHRONies (Calorie Restrictors on Optimal Nutrition) worldwide, and I have met quite a number of them. Despite their generally fabulous biochemical profile, I have never been seriously tempted to join their skinny ranks. I simply don't have the willpower or desire to live permanently on an extreme low-calorie diet.

So I was delighted to discover intermittent fasting, which involves eating fewer calories, but only some of the time. If the science was right, it offered the benefits of calorie restriction, but without the pain.

I set off around the US, meeting leading scientists who generously shared their research and ideas with me. It became clear that intermittent fasting was no fad. But it wouldn't be as easy as I'd originally hoped. As you'll see later in the book, there are many different forms of intermittent fasting. Some involve eating nothing for 24 hours or longer. Others involve a single, low-calorie meal once a day, every other day. I tried both but couldn't imagine doing either on a regular basis. I found it was simply too hard.

Instead I decided to create and test my own, modified version. Five days a week, I would eat normally; on the remaining two I would eat a quarter of my usual calorie intake (i.e. 600 calories).

I split the 600 calories in two – around 250 calories for breakfast and 350 calories for supper – effectively fasting for 12 hours at a stretch. I also decided to split my fasting days: I would fast on Mondays and Thursdays. I became my own experiment.

The programme, *Eat, Fast, Live Longer*, which detailed my adventures with what we were now calling the 5:2 diet, went out on the BBC during the London Olympics in August 2012. I expected it to be lost in the media frenzy that surrounded the Games, but instead it generated a frenzy of its own. The programme was watched by over 2.5 million people – a huge audience for *Horizon* – and hundreds of thousands more on YouTube. My Twitter account, @DrMichaelMosley, went into overdrive, my followers tripled; everyone wanted to try my version of intermittent fasting and they were all asking me what they should do.

The newspapers took up the story. Articles appeared in *The Times*, *The Daily Telegraph*, *The Daily Mail* and *The Mail on Sunday*. Before long, it was picked up by newspapers all over the world – in New York, Los Angeles, Paris, Madrid, Montreal, Islamabad and Delhi. Online groups were created, menus and experiences swapped, chat rooms started buzzing about fasting.

People began to stop me on the street and tell me how well they were doing on the 5:2 diet. They also emailed details of their experiences. Among those emails, a surprisingly large number were from doctors. Like me, they had initially been sceptical, but they had tried it for themselves, found that it worked and had begun suggesting it to their patients. They wanted information, menus, details of the scientific research to scrutinise. They wanted me to write a book. I hedged, procrastinated, then finally found a collaborator, Mimi Spencer, whom I liked and trusted and who has an in-depth knowledge of food. Which is how what you are reading came about.

Mimi's motivation: a female perspective

I started intermittent fasting on the day I was commissioned to write a feature for *The Times* about Michael's

Horizon programme. It was the first I'd heard of intermittent fasting, and the idea appealed immediately, even to a cynical soul who has spent two decades examining the curious acrobatics of the fashion industry, the beauty business and the diet trade.

I'd dabbled in diets before – show me a 40-something woman who hasn't – losing weight, then losing faith within weeks and piling it all back on. Though never overweight, I'd long been interested in dropping that reluctant half a stone or more – the pounds I picked up in pregnancy and somehow never lost. The diets I tried were always too hard to follow, too complicated to implement, too boring, too tough, too single-strand, too invasive, sucking the juice out of life and leaving you with the scraps. There was nothing I found that I could adopt and thread into the context of my life – as a mother, a working woman, a wife.

I've argued for years that dieting is a fool's game, doomed to fail because of the restrictions and deprivations imposed on an otherwise happy life, but this felt immediately different. The scientific evidence was extensive and compelling, and (crucially for me) the medical community was positive. The effects, for Michael and others, were impressive, startling even. In his *Horizon* documentary, Michael called it 'the beginning of something huge... which could radically transform the nation's health'. I couldn't resist. Nor could I conceive of a reason to wait.

In the two and a half years since I wrote *The Times* feature, I have remained a convert. An evangelist, actually. I'm still 'on' the Fast Diet now, following a 6:1 pattern, but I barely notice it. At the outset, I weighed 60kg (around nine and a half stone). At 5'7", my BMI was an OK 21.4. Today, as I write, I weigh 54kg (eight and a half stone) with a BMI of 19.4. That's a weight off. I feel light, lean and alive. Fasting has become part of my weekly life, something I do automatically without stressing about it.

These days, I have more energy, more bounce, clearer skin, a greater zest for life. And, it has to be said, new jeans (27-inch waist) and none of my annual bikini dread as summer approaches. But, perhaps more importantly, I know that there's a long-term gain. I'm doing the best for my body and my brain. It's an intimate revelation, but one worth sharing.

The Fast Diet: the potential, the promise

We know that for many people the standard diet advice simply does not work. The Fast Diet is a radical alternative. It has the potential to change the way we think about eating and weight loss.

- The Fast Diet demands we think not just about what we eat, but when we eat it

- There are no complicated rules to follow; the strategy is flexible, comprehensible and user-friendly

- There is no daily slog of calorie control – none of the boredom, frustration or serial deprivation that characterise conventional diet plans

- Yes, it involves fasting, but not as you know it; you won't 'starve' on any given day

- You can still enjoy the foods you love. Most of the time

- Once the weight is off, sticking to the basic programme will mean that it stays off

- Weight loss is only one benefit of the Fast Diet. The real dividend is the potential long-term health gains, cutting your risk of a range of diseases, including diabetes, heart disease and cancer

- You will soon come to understand that it is not just a diet. It is much more than that: it is a sustainable strategy for a healthy, long life

Now, you'll want to understand exactly how we can make these dramatic assertions. In the next chapter, Michael explains the science that makes the Fast Diet tick.

THE SCIENCE OF FASTING

For most animals out in the wild, periods of feast and famine are the norm. Our remote ancestors did not often eat four or five meals a day. Instead they would kill, gorge, lie around and then have to go for long periods of time without having anything to eat. Our bodies and our genes were forged in an environment of scarcity, punctuated by the occasional massive blow-out.

These days, of course, things are very different. We eat all the time. Fasting – the voluntary abstaining from eating food – is seen as a rather eccentric, not to mention unhealthy, thing to do. Most of us expect to eat at least three meals a day and have substantial snacks in between. In addition to the meals and the snacks, we also graze; a milky cappuccino here, the odd biscuit there, or maybe a smoothie because it's 'healthier'.

Once upon a time parents told their children not to eat between meals. Those times are long gone. Recent research in the US, which compared the eating habits of 28,000 children and 36,000 adults over the last 30 years, found that the amount of time spent between what the researchers coyly described as 'eating occasions' has fallen by an average of an hour. In other words, over the last few decades the amount of time we spend 'not eating' has dropped dramatically.[2] In the 1970s, people like my mother would go around four and a half hours without eating, while children like me would be expected to last about four hours between meals. Now it's down to three and a half hours for adults and three hours for children, and that doesn't include all the drinks and nibbles.

The idea that eating little and often is a 'good thing' has partly been driven by snack manufacturers and faddish diet books, but it has also had support from the medical establishment. Their argument is that it is better to eat lots of small meals because that way we are less likely to get hungry and gorge on high-fat junk. I can appreciate the argument, and there have been some studies that suggest there are health benefits to eating small meals regularly, as long as you don't simply end up eating more. Unfortunately, in the real world that's exactly what happens.

In the study I quoted above, they found that compared to 30 years ago, we not only eat around 180 calories a day more in snacks – much of it in the form of milky and fizzy drinks and smoothies – but we also eat more when it comes to our regular meals, up by an average of 120 calories a day.

In other words, snacking doesn't mean that we eat less at meal times; it just whets the appetite.

Do you need to eat lots of small meals to keep your metabolic rate high?

One of the other supposed benefits of eating lots of small meals is that this will increase your metabolic rate and help you lose weight. But is it true?

In a recent study researchers at the Institute for Clinical and Experimental Medicine in Prague decided to test this idea by feeding two groups of Type 2 diabetics meals with the same number of calories, but taken as either two or six meals a day.[3]

Both groups ate 1700 calories a day. The 'two meals a day' group ate their first meal between 6am and 10am and their next meal between 12pm and 4pm.

The 'snackers' ate their 1700 calories as six meals, spread out at regular intervals throughout the day.

Despite eating the same number of calories the 'two meals a day' group lost, on average, 1.4kg more than the snackers and about 1.5 inches more from around their waists.

Contrary to what you might expect, the volunteers eating their calories spread out over six meals a day felt less satisfied and hungrier than those sticking to the two meals. The lead scientist, Dr Kahleova, believes cutting down to two meals a day could also help people without diabetes who are trying to lose weight.

So, simply cutting out snacks and one meal a day could be an effective weight-loss strategy. Yet eating throughout the day is now so normal, so much the expected thing to do, that it is almost shocking to suggest there is value in doing the absolute opposite.

When I first started deliberately cutting back my calories two days a week I discovered some unexpected things about myself, my attitudes to food and about my beliefs.

- I discovered that I often eat when I don't need to. I do it because the food is there, because I am afraid that I will get hungry later, or simply from habit

- I assumed that when you get hungry it builds and builds until it becomes intolerable, and so you bury your face in a vat of ice cream. I found instead that hunger passes and once you have been really hungry you no longer fear it

- I thought that fasting would make me distractible, unable to concentrate. What I've discovered is that it sharpens my senses and my brain

- I wondered if I would feel faint for much of the time. It turns out that the body is incredibly adaptable and many athletes I've spoken to advocate training while fasting

- I feared it would be incredibly hard to do. It isn't

Why I got started

Although most of the great religions advocate fasting (the Sikhs are an exception, though they do allow fasting for medical reasons), I have always assumed that this was principally a way of testing yourself and your faith. I could see potential spiritual benefits but I was deeply sceptical about the physical benefits.

I have also had a number of body-conscious friends who, down the years, have tried to get me to fast, but I could never accept their explanation that the reason for doing so was 'to rest the liver' or 'to remove the toxins'. Neither explanation made any sense to a medically trained sceptic like me. I remember one friend telling me that after a couple of weeks of fasting his urine had turned black, proof that the toxins were leaving. I saw it as proof that he was an ignorant hippy and that whatever was going on inside his body as a result of fasting was extremely damaging. As I wrote earlier, what convinced me to try fasting was a combination of my own personal circumstances – in my mid-50s, high blood sugar, slightly overweight – and the emerging scientific evidence, which I list below.

That which does not kill us makes us stronger

There were a number of researchers who inspired me in

their different ways, but one who stands out is Professor Mark Mattson of the National Institute on Aging in Baltimore. Several years ago he wrote an article with Edward Calabrese in *New Scientist* magazine, 'When a little poison is good for you',[4] which really made me sit up and think.

'A little poison is good for you' is a colourful way of describing the theory of hormesis – the idea that when a human, or indeed any other creature, is exposed to a stress or toxin it can toughen them up. Hormesis is not just a variant of 'join the army and it will make a man of you'; it is now a well-accepted explanation in biology of how things operate at the cellular level.

Take, for example, something as simple as exercise. When you run or pump iron, what you are actually doing is damaging your muscles, causing small tears and rips. If you don't completely overdo it, then your body responds by doing repairs and in the process makes the muscles stronger.

Thinking or having to make decisions can also be stressful, yet there is good evidence that challenging yourself intellectually is good for your brain, and the reason it is good is that it produces changes in brain cells that are similar to the changes you see in muscle cells after exercise. The right sort of stress keeps us younger and smarter.

Vegetables are another example of the power of hormesis. We all know that we should eat lots of fruit and vegetables because they are chock full of antioxidants – and antioxidants are great because they mop up the dangerous free radicals that roam our bodies doing harm.

The trouble with this widely accepted explanation of how fruit and vegetables 'work' is that it is almost certainly wrong, or at least incomplete. The levels of antioxidants in fruits and vegetables are far too low to have the profound effects they clearly do. In addition, the attempts to extract antioxidants from plants and then give them to us in a concentrated form, as a health-inducing supplement, have been unconvincing when tested in long-term trials. Betacarotene, when you get it in the form of a carrot, is undoubtedly good for you. When they took betacarotene out of the carrot and gave it as a supplement to patients with cancer, it actually seemed to make them worse.

If we look through the prism of hormesis at the way vegetables work in our bodies, we can see that the reasons for their benefits may be quite different.

Consider this apparent paradox: bitterness is often associated in the wild with poisons, something to be avoided. Plants produce a huge range of so-called phytochemicals and some of them act as natural pesticides, to keep mammals like us from eating them. The fact that they taste bitter is a clear warning signal: keep away. So there are good evolutionary reasons why we should dislike and avoid bitter-tasting foods. Yet some of the vegetables that are particularly good for us, such as cabbage, cauliflower, broccoli and other members of the brassica family, are so bitter that even as adults many of us struggle to love them.

The resolution to this paradox is that these vegetables taste bitter because they contain chemicals that are potentially poisonous. The reason they don't harm us is that these chemicals are present in them at low doses that are not toxic. Rather, they activate stress responses and switch on genes that protect and repair.

Once you start looking at the world in this way, you realise that many activities we initially find stressful – like eating bitter vegetables, going for a run, or intermittent fasting – are far from harmful. The challenge itself seems to be part of the benefit. The fact that prolonged starvation is clearly very bad for you does not imply that short periods of intermittent fasting must be a little bit bad for you. Indeed the reverse is true.

This point was vividly made to me by Professor Valter Longo, director of the University of Southern California's Longevity Institute. His research is mainly into the study of why we age, particularly concerning approaches that reduce the risk of developing age-related diseases such as cancer and diabetes.

I went to see Valter, not just because he is a world expert, but also because he had kindly agreed to act as my fasting mentor and buddy, to help inspire and guide me through my first experience of fasting.

Valter has been studying fasting for many years, and he is a keen adherent of it. He lives by his research and thrives on the sort of low-protein, high-vegetable diet that his grandparents enjoy in southern Italy. Perhaps not coincidentally, his grandparents live in a part of Italy that has an extraordinarily high concentration of long-lived people.

As well as following a fairly strict diet, Valter skips lunch to keep his weight down. Beyond this, once every six months or so, he does a prolonged fast that lasts several days. Tall, slim, energetic, he is an inspiring poster boy for would-be fasters.

The main reason he is so enthusiastic about fasting is that his research, and that of others, has demonstrated the extraordinary range of measurable health benefits that you get from doing it. Going without food for even quite short periods of time switches on a number of 'repair genes', which, as he explained, can confer long-term benefits. 'There is a lot of initial evidence to suggest that temporary periodic fasting can induce long-lasting changes that can be beneficial against ageing and diseases,' he told me. 'You take a person, you fast them, after 24 hours everything is revolutionised. And even if you took a cocktail of drugs, very potent drugs, you will never even get close to what fasting does. The beauty of fasting is that it's all co-ordinated.'

Fasting and longevity

Most of the early long-term studies on the benefits of fasting were done with rodents. They also gave us important insights into the molecular mechanisms that underpin fasting.

In one early study from 1945, mice were fasted for either one day in four, one day in three or one day in two. The researchers found that the fasted mice lived longer than a control group, and that the more they fasted the longer they lived. They also found that, unlike calorie-restricted mice, the fasted mice were not physically stunted.[5]

Since then numerous studies have confirmed, at least in rodents, the value of fasting. Not only does fasting extend their lifespan, but it also increases their 'health-span', the amount of time they live without chronic age-related diseases. Post-mortems on rodents that have been calorie-restricted show they display far fewer signs of cancer, heart disease or neurodegeneration.

A recent article in the prestigious science journal *Nature* points to the wealth of research on the benefits of fasting while at the same time noting sadly that so far 'these insights have made hardly a dent in human medicine'.[6]

But why does fasting help? What is the mechanism?

Valter has access to his own supply of genetically

engineered mice, known as dwarf or Laron mice, which he was keen to show me. These mice, though small, hold the record for longevity extension in a mammal. In other words, they live for an astonishingly long time.

The average mouse doesn't live that long, perhaps two years. Laron mice can live twice that, many for over four years when they are also calorie-restricted. In a human, that would be the equivalent of reaching almost 170.

The fascinating thing about Laron mice is not just their longevity, but the fact that they stay healthy for most of their very long lives. They simply don't seem to be prone to diabetes or cancer, and when they die, more often than not, it is of natural causes. Valter told me that on autopsy they are often unable to find a cause of death. They just seem to drop dead.

The reason these mice are so small and so long-lived is that they are genetically engineered so that their bodies do not respond to a hormone called IGF-1, Insulin-Like Growth Factor 1. IGF-1, as its name implies, has growth-promoting effects on almost every cell in your body. It keeps your cells constantly active. You need adequate levels of IGF-1 and other growth factors when you are young and growing, but high levels later in life appear to lead to accelerated ageing and cancer. As Valter put it, it's like driving along with your foot flat down on the accelerator, pushing the car to continue to perform all the time. 'Imagine, instead of occasionally taking your car to the garage and changing parts and pieces, you simply kept on driving it and driving it and driving it. Well, the car, of course, is going to break down.'

Valter's work is focused on trying to figure out how you can go on driving as much as possible, and as fast as possible, while enjoying life. He thinks the answer is periodic fasting. Because one of the ways fasting works is by making your body reduce the amount of IGF-1 it produces.

The evidence that IGF-1 plays a key role in many of the diseases of ageing comes not just from rodents like the Laron mice but also from humans. For the last seven years, Valter has been studying villagers in Ecuador with a genetic defect, a syndrome also called Laron. This is an extremely rare condition which affects fewer than 350 people in the world. People with Laron syndrome have bodies which don't seem to be able to respond to IGF-1. There's a specific mutation in the growth hormone receptor, causing a deficiency that is very similar to that in the Laron mouse.

The villagers with Laron syndrome are normally quite short; many are less than four feet tall. The thing that is most surprising about them, however, is that, like the Laron mice, they simply don't seem to develop common diseases like diabetes and cancer. In fact, Valter says that, though they have been studied for many years, there is not a single case he has come across of someone with Laron dying of cancer. Yet their relatives, who live in the same household but who don't have Laron syndrome, get cancer like everybody else.

Disappointingly, for anyone hoping that IGF-1 will provide the secrets of immortality, people with Laron syndrome, unlike the mice, are not exceptionally long-lived. They certainly lead long lives, but not super-long lives. Valter thinks one reason for this may be that they tend to enjoy life rather than worry about their lifestyle. 'They smoke, eat a high-calorie diet, and then they look at me and they say, "Oh it doesn't matter, I'm immune."'

Valter thinks they prefer the idea of living as they want and dying at 85, rather than living more carefully and perhaps going beyond 100. He would like to persuade some of them to take on a healthy lifestyle and see what happens, but knows he wouldn't live long enough to see the outcome.

Fasting and repair genes

As well as reducing circulating levels of IGF-1, fasting also appears to switch on a number of repair genes. The reason this happens is not fully understood, but the evolutionary argument goes something like this. As long as we have plenty of food, our bodies are mainly interested in growing, having sex and reproducing. Nature has no long-term plans for us. She does not invest in our old age. Once we have reproduced we become disposable.

So what happens if you decide to fast? Well, the body's initial reaction is one of shock. Signals go to the brain reminding you that you are hungry, urging you to go out and find something to eat. But you resist. The body now decides that the reason you are not eating as much and as frequently as you usually do must be because you are now in a famine situation. In the past this would have been quite normal.

In a famine situation there is no point in expending energy on growth or sex. Instead the wisest thing the body can do is spend its precious store of energy on repair, trying to keep you in reasonable shape until the good times return once more. The result is that, as well as removing its foot from the accelerator, your body takes itself along to the cellular equivalent of a garage. There, all the little gene mechanics are ordered to start doing some of the urgent maintenance tasks that have been put off till now.

One of the things that calorie restriction does, for example, is switch on a process called autophagy.[7] Autophagy, meaning 'self eat', is a process by which the body breaks down and recycles old and tired cells; just as with a car, it is important to get rid of damaged or ageing parts if you are going to keep things in good working order.

Intermittent fasting and stem cell regeneration

Fasting not only helps clear out damaged old cells but can also spark the production of new ones. In a particularly fascinating study published in June 2014, Valter and his colleagues showed, for the first time, that fasting can switch on stem cells and regenerate the immune system.[8]

Stem cells are cells that, when activated, can grow into almost any other cell. They can become brain, liver, heart tissue, whatever. The study findings are exciting because as we age our immune system tends to get weaker. Being able to create new white cells and a more powerful immune system will not only keep infections at bay but may also reduce your risk of developing cancer; mutating cells that could turn into a cancer are normally destroyed by the immune system long before they can escape and multiply.

There have been claims that fasting can harm your immune system and, initially, Valter's studies seemed to support this view, as he explains, 'When you starve, your system tries to save energy, and one of the things it can do to save energy is to recycle a lot of the immune cells that are not needed, especially those that may be damaged. What we started noticing in both our human work and animal work is that the white blood cell count goes down with prolonged fasting.'

Clearly in the long run this would be harmful, as a fall in white blood cells would make you more vulnerable to infections and cancers. But, as we have seen with hormesis, just because something is bad for you when pushed to the extreme, that does not mean it is bad when done in moderation.

Valter discovered, to his considerable surprise, that if you do a short fast and then eat, you get a rebound effect, with the creation of new, more active cells. 'We could not have predicted,' he said, 'that fasting would have such a remarkable effect.'

It seems that fasting not only clears out the old, damaged white blood cells and lowers levels of IGF-1, but also reduces the activity of a gene called PKA. PKA produces an enzyme that normally acts like a brake on regeneration.

'PKA is the key gene that needs to be shut down in order for stem cells to switch into regenerative mode,' Valter says.

Intermittent fasting seems to give the 'okay' for stem cells to go ahead and begin proliferating. This research certainly suggests that if your immune system is not as effective as it was (either because you are older or because you have had a medical treatment such as chemotherapy), then periods of intermittent fasting may help regenerate it.

Michael experiences a four-day fast

Valter thinks that the majority of people with a BMI

over 25 would benefit from fasting, but he also thinks that if you plan to do it for more than a day it should be done in a proper centre. As he put it, 'a prolonged fast is an extreme intervention. If it's done well, it can be very powerful in your favour. If it's done improperly, it can be very powerful against you.' With a fast lasting several days, you also get a drop in blood pressure and some fairly profound metabolic reprogramming. Some people faint. It's not common but it happens.

As Valter pointed out, the first time you try prolonged fasting it can be a bit of a struggle. 'Our bodies are used to high levels of glucose and high levels of insulin, so it takes time to adapt. But then eventually it's not that hard.'

I wasn't keen to hear 'eventually', but I knew as soon as I met Valter that I would have to give it a go. It was a challenge, and one I thought I could win. Brain against stomach. No contest.

I had recently had my IGF-1 levels measured and they were high. Not super-high, as he kindly put it, but at the top end of the range (my levels of IGF-1 or somatomedin-C, as it's also known, were 28.0nmol/l. The healthy range is 11.3–30.9nmol/l).

High levels of IGF-1 are associated with a range of cancers, among them prostate cancer which had troubled my father. Would a four-day fast change anything?

Valter had told me that once I got through the first couple of tough days, I would start to feel the effects of a rush of what he termed 'wellbeing chemicals'. Even better, the next time I fasted it would be easier because my body and brain would have a memory of it and understand what I was going through.

Having decided that I would try an extended fast, my next decision was how harsh to make it. A number of different countries have a tradition of fasting. The Russians seem to prefer it tough. For them, a fast consists of nothing but water, cold showers and exercise. The Germans, on the other hand, prefer their fasts to be considerably gentler. Go to a fasting clinic in Germany and you will probably be fed around 200 calories a day in comfortable surroundings. I wanted to see results, so I went for a British comprom-ise. I would eat 25 calories a day, no cold showers and just try working as normal.

So on a warm Monday evening, I enjoyed my last meal, a filling dinner of steak, chips and salad washed down with beer. I felt a certain trepidation as I realised that for the next four days I would be drinking nothing but water, sugarless black tea and coffee, and one measly cup of low-calorie soup a day.

Despite what I'd read and been told, before I began my fast I secretly feared that hunger would grow and grow, gnawing away inside me until I finally gave in and ran amok in a cake shop. The first 24 hours were quite tough, just as Valter had predicted, but as he had also predicted things got better, not worse. Yes, there were hunger pangs, sometimes quite distracting, but if I kept busy they went away.

During the first 24 hours of a fast, there are some quite profound changes going on inside the body. Within a few hours, glucose circulating in the blood is consumed. If that's not being replaced by food then the body turns to glycogen, a stable form of glucose that is stored in the muscles and liver.

Only when that's gone does it really switch on fat burning. What actually happens is that fatty acids are broken down in the liver, resulting in the production of something called ketone bodies. The brain uses these ketone bodies as a source of energy, instead of glucose.

The first two days of a fast can be uncomfortable because your body and brain are having to cope with the switch from using glucose and glycogen as a fuel to using ketone bodies. The body is not used to them so you can get headaches, though I didn't. You may find it hard to sleep. I didn't. The biggest problem I had with fasting is hard to put into words; it was sometimes just feeling 'uncomfortable'. I can't really describe it more accurately than that. I didn't feel faint; I just felt out of place.

I did, occasionally, feel hungry, but most of the time I was surprisingly cheerful. By day three the feel-good hormones had come to my rescue.

By Friday, day four, I was almost disappointed that it was ending. Almost. Despite Valter's warning that it would be unwise to gorge immediately on breaking a fast, I got myself a plate of bacon and eggs and settled down to eat. After a few mouthfuls I was full. I really didn't need any more and in fact skipped lunch.

That afternoon I was tested again and discovered I had lost just under three pounds of body weight, a significant portion of which was fat. I was also happy to see that my blood glucose levels had fallen substantially and that my IGF-1 levels, which had been at the top end of the recommended range, had gone right down. In fact, they had almost halved. This was all good news. I had lost some fat, my blood results were looking good, and I had learnt that I could control my hunger. Valter was extremely pleased with these changes, particularly the fall in IGF-1 that he said would significantly reduce my risk of cancer. But he also warned me that if I went back to my old lifestyle these changes would not be permanent.

Valter's research points towards the fact that high levels of protein, the amounts found in a typical western diet, help keep IGF-1 levels high. I knew that there is protein in foods like meat and fish, but I was surprised that there is so much in milk. I used to like drinking a skinny latte most mornings. I had the illusion that because it is made with skimmed milk it is healthy. Unfortunately, though low in fat, a large latte comes in at around 11g of protein. And Valter recommends that you don't eat more than 0.8g of protein per kg of body weight per day. For someone like me, that would be around 64g a day. The lattes would have to go.

Fasting and weight loss

I did the four-day fast, as described above, mainly because I was curious. I would not recommend it as a weight-loss regime because it is completely unsustainable. Unless they combine it with a vigorous exercise regime, people who go on prolonged fasts lose muscle as well as fat. Then, when they stop, as they must eventually do, the risk is they will pile the weight right back on.

Fortunately, less drastic, intermittent fasting – the subject of this book – leads to steady and sustainable weight loss and does not cause muscle loss.

Alternate Day Fasting

One of the most extensively studied forms of short-term fasting is Alternate Day Fasting (ADF). As its name implies, it means you get no food, or relatively little food, every other day.

Dr Krista Varady of the University of Illinois at Chicago has done a lot of the more recent studies on ADF.

Krista is slim, charming and very amusing. We first met in an old-fashioned American diner where I guiltily ate burgers and fries while Krista told me about the work she has been carrying out with human volunteers.[9] The version of ADF she has been testing is one where on fasting days volunteers are allowed 25% of their normal energy needs, so men are allowed around 600 calories a day, women 500 calories a day. On Fast Days they eat all their calories in one go, at lunch. On their feed days they are asked to consume 125% of their normal energy needs.

Krista has been surprised to find that, even when they are allowed to, people don't go crazy on their feed days. 'I thought when I started running these trials that people would eat 175% the next day; they'd just fully compensate and wouldn't lose any weight. But most people eat around 110%, just slightly over what they usually eat. I haven't measured it yet, but I think it involves stomach size, how far that can expand out. Because eating almost twice the amount of food that you normally eat is actually pretty difficult. You can do it over time; people that are obese, their stomachs get bigger to accommodate, you know, 5000 calories a day. But just to do it right off is actually pretty difficult.'

In her earlier studies, subjects were asked to stick to a low-fat diet, but what Krista wanted to know was whether ADF would also work if her subjects were allowed to eat a typical American high-fat diet. So she asked 33 obese volunteers, most of them women, to go on ADF for eight weeks. Before starting, the volunteers were divided into two groups. One group was put on a low-fat diet, eating low-fat cheeses and dairies, very lean meats and a lot of fruit and vegetables. The other group was allowed to eat high-fat lasagnes, pizza, the sort of diet a typical American might consume. Americans consume somewhere between

35 and 45% fat in their diet.

As Krista explained, the results were unexpected. The researchers and volunteers had assumed that the people on the low-fat diet would lose more weight than those on the high-fat diet. But, if anything, it was the other way around. The volunteers on the high-fat diet lost an average of 5.6kg, while those on the low-fat diet lost 4.2kg. They both lost about seven centimetres around their waists.

Krista thinks that the main reason this happened was compliance. The volunteers randomised to the high-fat diet were more likely to stick to it than those on the low-fat diet simply because they found it a lot more palatable. And it wasn't just weight loss. Both groups saw impressive falls in low-density lipoprotein (LDL) cholesterol, the bad cholesterol, and in blood pressure. This meant that they had reduced their risk of cardiovascular disease, of having a heart attack or stroke.

Krista doesn't want to encourage people to binge on rubbish. She would much rather that people on ADF ate healthily, increased their fruit and vegetable intake, and generally ate less. The trouble is, as she pointed out rather exasperatedly, doctors have been encouraging people to embrace a healthy lifestyle for decades, and not enough of us are doing it. She thinks dieticians should take into account what people actually do rather than what we would like them to do.

One other significant benefit of intermittent fasting is that you don't seem to lose muscle, which you would on a normal calorie-restricted regime. Krista herself is not sure why that is and wants to do further research.

The two-day fast

If you want to lose weight fast, then ADF is an effective, scientifically proven way to do it. The problem I had with ADF, which is why I personally am not so keen on it, is that you have to do it every other day.

In my experience this can be socially inconvenient as well as emotionally demanding. There is no pattern to your week and other people, friends and family, find it hard to keep track of when your fast and feed days are. Unlike Krista's subjects, I was not particularly overweight to start with, so I also worried about losing too much weight too rapidly. That is why, having tried ADF for a short while, I decided to cut back to fasting two days a week.

I now have my own experience of this to fall back on (see page 74), together with the experiences of thousands of others who have written to me over the last two years.

But what trials have been done on two-day fasts in humans? Well, Dr Michelle Harvie, a dietician based at the Genesis Breast Cancer Prevention Centre at the Wythenshawe Hospital in Manchester, has done a number of studies assessing the effects of a two-day fast on female volunteers.

In a recent study, she divided 115 women into three groups. One group was asked to stick to a 1500-calorie Mediterranean diet, and was also encouraged to avoid high-fat foods and alcohol.[10] Another group was asked to eat normally five days a week, but to eat a 650-calorie, low-carbohydrate diet on the other two days. A final group was asked to avoid carbohydrates for two days a week, but was otherwise not calorie-restricted.

After three months, the women on the two-day diets had lost an average of 3.6kg of fat, which was almost twice as much as the full-time dieters, who had lost an average of 2kg of fat. Insulin resistance had also improved significantly in the two-day diet groups (see more on insulin on page 60).

Those who stuck with the two-day diet for six months lost an average of 7.7kg and three inches from their waists. Some lost over 20kg.

The focus of Michelle's work is trying to reduce breast cancer risk through dietary interventions. Being obese and having high levels of insulin resistance are both risk factors. On the Genesis website (www.genesisuk.org), she points out that they have been studying Intermittent Fasting at the Genesis Breast Cancer Prevention Centre, University Hospital of South Manchester NHS Foundation Trust, for over eight years and that their research has shown that cutting down on your calories for two days a week gives the same benefits, possibly more, than by going on a normal calorie-reduced diet. 'To date, our research has concluded that intermittent diets appear to be a safe, viable, alternative approach to weight loss and maintaining a lower weight, in comparison to daily dieting.'

Another, more recent study, looked at the effects of a two-day diet on the mood of those taking part.[11]

In this study, from Malaysia, 32 healthy males with an average age of 60 were randomly allocated either a Sunnah fast (a Muslim fast), which meant cutting their calories on a Monday and a Thursday, or to a control group. They were then followed for three months.

Their mood was assessed using something called, 'The Profile of Mood States' questionnaire. The researchers found that not only did the intermittent fasting group lose far more fat than the control group, but also that they felt much better on it. The researchers found that those doing intermittent fasting reported: 'Significant decreases in tension, anger, confusion and total mood disturbance and improvements in vigour.'

On an anecdotal level I have heard very good things from those who have tried intermittent fasting. Many people find it surprisingly easy, others struggle, but generally things improve after the first couple of weeks. As one faster says, 'I used to have mood swings as well as headaches; it does pass as you get used to this new way of eating, I found by week six it had become part of my routine.'

Is it just calories?

If you eat 500 or 600 calories two days a week and don't significantly overcompensate during the rest of the week, then you will lose weight in a steady fashion.

I recently came across one particularly fascinating study, though, suggesting that *when* you eat can be almost as important as *what* you eat.

In this study, scientists from the Salk Institute for Biological Studies took two groups of mice and fed them a high-fat diet.[12] The mice got exactly the same amount of food to eat, the only difference being that one group of mice was allowed to eat whenever they wanted, nibbling away when they were in the mood, rather like we do, while the other group of mice had to eat their food in an eight-hour time period. This meant that there were 16 hours of the day in which they were, involuntarily, fasting.

After 100 days, there were some truly dramatic differences between the two groups of mice. The mice that nibbled away at their fatty food had developed high cholesterol, high blood glucose and had liver damage. The mice that had been forced to fast for 16 hours a day put on far less weight (28% less) and suffered much less liver damage, despite having eaten exactly the same amount and quality of food. They also had lower levels of chronic inflammation, which suggests they had a reduced risk of a number of diseases, including heart disease, cancer, stroke and Alzheimer's.

The Salk researchers' explanation for this is that all the time you are eating your insulin levels are elevated and your body is stuck in fat-storing mode (see the discussion of insulin on page 60). Only after a few hours of fasting is your body able to turn off the 'fat-storing' and turn on the 'fat-burning' mechanisms. So if you are a mouse and you are continually nibbling, your body will just continue making and storing fat, resulting in obesity and liver damage.

I think there is strong evidence that fasting offers multiple health benefits, as well as helping to achieve weight loss. I had been aware of some of these claims before I got really interested in fasting and, though initially sceptical, I was converted by the sheer weight of evidence.

But there was one area of study that was a complete surprise: research showing how fasting can improve mood and protect the brain from dementia and cognitive decline. This, for me, was something completely new, unexpected, and hugely exciting.

Fasting and the brain

The brain, as Woody Allen once said, is my second favourite organ. I might even put it first, as without it nothing else would function. The human brain, around three pounds of pinkish greyish gunk with the consistency of tapioca, has been described as the most complex object in the known universe. It allows us to build, write poetry, dominate the planet and even understand ourselves, something no other creature has succeeded in doing.

It is also an extremely efficient energy-saving machine, doing all that complicated thinking and making sure our bodies are functioning properly while using the same amount of energy as a 25-watt light bulb. The fact that our brains are normally so flexible and adaptable makes it even more tragic when they go wrong. I am aware that as I get older my memory has become more fallible. I've compensated by using a range of memory tricks I've picked up over the years, but even so I find myself occasionally struggling to remember names and dates.

Far worse than this, however, is the fear that one day I may lose my mind entirely, perhaps developing some form of dementia. Obviously I want to preserve my brain in as good a shape as possible and for as long as possible. Fortunately fasting seems to offer significant protection.

The man I went to discuss my brain with was Professor Mark Mattson.

Mark Mattson, a professor of neuroscience at the National Institute on Aging, is one of the most revered scientists in his field: the study of the ageing brain. I find his work genuinely inspiring – suggesting, as it does, that fasting can help combat diseases like Alzheimer's, as well as other forms of dementia and memory loss.

Although I could have taken a taxi to his office, I chose to walk. I'm a fan of walking. It not only burns calories, it also improves the mood, and it may also help retain your memory. Normally as we get older our brain shrinks, but one study found that in regular walkers the hippocampus, an area of the brain essential for memory, actually expanded.[13] Regular walkers have brains that in MRI scans look, on average, two years younger than the brains of those who are sedentary.

Mark, who studies Alzheimer's, lost his own father to dementia. He told me that although it didn't directly motivate him to go into this particular line of research – when he started work on Alzheimer's disease his father had not yet been diagnosed – but it did give him insight.

Alzheimer's affects around 26 million people worldwide and the problem will grow as the population ages. New approaches are desperately needed because the tragedy of Alzheimer's disease and other forms of dementia is that once you're diagnosed it may be possible to delay, but not prevent, the inevitable deterioration. You are likely to get progressively worse to the point where you need constant care for many years. By the end you may not even recognise the faces of those you once loved.

Can fasting make you clever?

Just as Valter Longo had, Mark took me off to see some mice. Like Valter's mice, Mark's mice are genetically engineered, but they have been modified to make them more vulnerable to Alzheimer's. The mice I saw were in a maze, which they had to navigate in order to find food. Some of the mice perform this task with relative ease; others get disorientated and confused. This task, and others like it, are designed to reveal signs that the mice are developing memory problems; a mouse that is struggling will quickly forget which arm of the maze it has already travelled down.

The genetically engineered Alzheimer's mice will, if put on a normal diet, quickly develop dementia. By the time they are a year old, the equivalent of middle age in humans, they normally have obvious learning and memory problems. The animals put on an intermittent fast, something Mark prefers to call 'intermittent energy restriction', often go up to 20 months without any detectable signs of dementia.[14] They only really start deteriorating towards the end of their lives. In humans that would be the equivalent of developing signs of Alzheimer's at the age of 80 rather than at 50. I know which I would prefer.

Disturbingly, when these mice are put on a typical junk-food diet, they go downhill much earlier than even normally fed mice. 'We put mice on a high-fat and high-fructose diet,' Mark said, 'and that has a dramatic effect;

the animals have an earlier onset of the learning and memory problems, more accumulation of amyloid and more problems with finding their way in a maze test.'

In other words, junk food makes these mice fat and stupid.

One of the key changes that occur in the brains of Mark's fasting mice is increased production of a protein called brain-derived neurotrophic factor. BDNF has been shown to stimulate stem cells to turn into new nerve cells in the hippocampus. As I mentioned earlier, this is a part of the brain that is essential for normal learning and memory.

But why should the hippocampus grow in response to fasting? Mark points out that from an evolutionary perspective it makes sense. After all, the times when you need to be smart and on the ball are when there's not a lot of food lying around. 'If an animal is in an area where there's limited food resources, it's important that they are able to remember where food is, remember where hazards are, predators and so on. We think that people in the past who were able to respond to hunger with increased cognitive ability had a survival advantage.'

We don't know for sure if humans grow new brain cells in response to fasting; to be absolutely certain researchers would need to put volunteers on an intermittent fast and then kill them, take their brains out and look for signs of new neural growth. It seems unlikely that many would volunteer for such a project. But what they are doing is a study where volunteers fast and then MRI scans are used to see if the size of their hippocampi change over time.

As we have seen, these techniques have been used in humans to show that regular exercise, such as walking, increases the size of the hippocampus. Hopefully similar studies will show that two days a week of intermittent fasting is good for learning and memory. On a purely anecdotal level, and using a sample size of one, it seems to work. Before starting the Fast Diet, I did a sophisticated memory test online. Two months in I repeated the test and my performance had, indeed, improved. If you are interested in doing something similar then I suggest you go to www.cognitivefun.net/test/2. Do let us know how you get on.

Fasting and mood

One of the things that Professor Valter Longo and others told me before I began my four-day fast was that it would be tough initially, but that after a while I would start to feel more cheerful, which was indeed what happened. Similarly, I was surprised to discover how positive I have felt while doing intermittent fasting. I expected to feel tired and crabby on my fasting days, but not at all. So is this simply a psychological effect, that people who do intermittent fasting and lose weight feel good about themselves, or are there also chemical changes that are influencing mood?

According to Professor Mark Mattson, one of the reasons people find intermittent fasting relatively easy to do may be due to its effects on BDNF. BDNF not only seems to protect the brain against the ravages of dementia and age-related mental decline, but it may also improve your mood.

There have been a number of studies going back many years that suggest rising levels of BDNF have an anti-depressant effect, at least in rodents. In one study, they injected BDNF directly into the brains of rats and found this had similar effects to repeated use of a standard anti-depressant.[15] Another paper found that electric shock therapy, which is known to be effective in severe depression, seems to work, at least in part, because it stimulates the production of higher levels of BDNF.[16]

Mark Mattson believes that within a few weeks of starting a two-day-a-week fasting regime, BDNF levels will start to rise, suppressing anxiety and elevating mood. He doesn't currently have the human data to fully support this claim, but he is doing trials on volunteers which involve, among other things, collecting regular samples of cerebrospinal fluid (the liquid that bathes the brain) in order to measure the changes that occur during intermittent fasts. This is not a trial for the faint-hearted as it requires regular spinal taps, but as Mark pointed out to me, many of his volunteers are already undergoing early signs of cognitive change, so they are extremely motivated.

Mark is keen to study and promote the benefits of intermittent fasting as he is genuinely worried about the likely effects of the current obesity epidemic on our brains and our society. He also thinks that if you are considering intermittent fasting you should get going sooner rather than later: 'The age-related cognitive decline in Alzheimer's disease, the events that are occurring in the brain at the level of the nerve cells and the molecules in the nerve cells, those changes are occurring very early, probably decades before the subject starts to have learning and memory problems. That's why it's critical to start dietary regimes early on, when people are young or middle-aged, so that they can slow down the development of these processes in the brain and live to be 90 with their brain functioning perfectly well.'

Like Mark, I'm convinced the human brain benefits from short periods abstaining from food. This is an exciting and fast-emerging area of research that many will watch with great interest. Beyond the brain, though, intermittent fasting also has measurable, beneficial effects on other areas of the body – on your heart, on your blood profile, on your risk of cancer. And that's where we'll turn now.

Fasting and the heart

One of the main reasons I decided to try fasting was that tests had suggested I was heading for serious problems with my cardiovascular system. Nothing has happened yet, but the warning signs were flashing amber. The tests showed that my blood levels of LDL (low-density lipoprotein, the 'bad' cholesterol) were disturbingly high, as were the levels of my fasting glucose.

To measure 'fasting glucose' you have to fast overnight, then give a sample of blood. The normal, desirable range is 3.9–5.8mmol/l. Mine was 7.3mmol/l. Diabetic, but not yet dangerously high. There are many reasons why you should do all you can to avoid becoming a diabetic, not least the fact that it dramatically increases your risk of having a heart attack or stroke.

Fasting glucose is an important thing to measure because it is an indicator that all may not be well with your insulin levels.

Insulin – the fat-making hormone

Insulin is a hormone that has a similar molecular structure to IGF-1, and like IGF-1 it tends to increase cell turnover and reduce autophagy (clearing up of old cells). But insulin is best known as a hormone that regulates blood sugar. When we eat food, particularly food rich in carbohydrates, our blood glucose levels rise and the pancreas starts to churn out insulin. Glucose is the main fuel that our cells use for energy, but high levels of glucose circulating in the blood are toxic to your cells. The job of insulin is to regulate blood glucose levels, ensuring that they are neither too high nor too low. It normally does this with great precision. The problem comes when the pancreas gets overloaded.

Insulin is a sugar controller; it aids the extraction of glucose from blood and then stores it in places like your liver or muscles in a stable form called glycogen, to be used when and if it is needed. What is less commonly known is that insulin is also a fat controller. It inhibits something called lipolysis, the release of stored body fat. At the same time, it forces fat cells to take up and store fat from your blood. Insulin makes you fat. High levels lead to increased fat storage, low levels to fat depletion.

The trouble with constantly eating lots of sugary, carbohydrate-rich foods and drinks, as we increasingly do, is that this requires the release of more and more insulin to deal with the glucose surge. Up to a point, your pancreas will cope by simply pumping out ever-larger quantities of insulin. This leads to greater fat deposition and also increases the risk of cancer. Naturally enough, this can't go on for ever. If you continue to produce ever-larger quantities of insulin, your cells will eventually rebel and become resistant to its effects. It's rather like shouting at your children; you can keep escalating things, but after a certain point they will simply stop listening.

Eventually the cells stop responding to insulin; your blood glucose levels now stay permanently high and you will find you have joined the 285 million people around the world who have Type 2 diabetes. It is a massive and rapidly growing problem worldwide. Over the last 20 years, numbers have risen almost tenfold and there is no obvious sign that this trend is slowing.

Diabetes is associated with an increased risk of heart attack, stroke, impotence, going blind and losing your extremities due to poor circulation. It is also associated with brain shrinkage and dementia. Not a pretty picture.

One way to prevent the downward spiral into diabetes is to cut back on the carbohydrates and instead start eating more vegetables and fat, since these foods do not lead to such big spikes in blood glucose. Nor do they have such a dramatic effect on insulin levels. The other way is to try intermittent fasting.

How intermittent fasting affects insulin sensitivity and diabetes

In a study from 2005, eight healthy young men were asked to fast every other day, 20 hours a day, for two weeks.[17] On their fasting days they were allowed to eat until 10pm, then not eat again until 6pm the following evening. They were also asked to eat heartily the rest of the time to make sure they did not lose any weight.

The idea behind the experiment was to test the so-called 'thrifty hypothesis', the idea that since we evolved at a time of feast and famine the best way to eat is to mimic those times. At the end of the two weeks, there were no changes in the volunteers' weight or body-fat composition, which is what the researchers had intended. There was, however, a big change in their insulin sensitivity. In other words, after just two weeks of intermittent fasting, the same amount of circulating insulin now had a much greater effect on the volunteers' ability to store glucose or break down fat.

The researchers wrote jubilantly that, 'by subjecting healthy men to cycles of feast and famine we changed their metabolic status for the better'. They also added that, 'to our knowledge this is the first study in humans in which an increased insulin action on whole body glucose uptake and adipose tissue lipolysis has been obtained by means of intermittent fasting.'

One of the ways that intermittent fasting seems to improve insulin sensitivity is by forcing the body to break down fat cells and use the fat as an energy source. Researchers at the Intermountain Heart Institute in Utah reported at a recent meeting of the American Diabetes Association that after 10 to 12 hours without food the body starts looking for new energy sources. At the same time it starts drawing LDL cholesterol from cells, possibly using it as a fuel.

Dr Benjamin Horne, director of the Institute, says that because fat cells are a major contributor to insulin resistance (when the body stops responding to insulin), breaking down fat cells may reduce the risk of diabetes developing. Short-term fasting also makes the cells of the body go into a self-protection mode in which they become resensitised to insulin.

'Although fasting may protect against diabetes,' Dr Horne cautions, 'it's important to keep in mind that these results are not instantaneous. It takes time. How long and how often people should fast for health benefits are additional questions we're just beginning to examine.'

I don't know what impact intermittent fasting has had on my insulin sensitivity – it's a test that is hard to do and extremely expensive – but what I do know is that the effects on my blood sugar have been spectacular. Before I started fasting, my blood glucose level was 7.3 mmol/l, well above the acceptable range of 3.9 – 5.8 mmol/l. The last time I had my level measured it was 5.0 mmol/l, still a bit high but well within the normal range.

This is an incredibly impressive response. My doctor, who was preparing to put me on medication, was astonished at such a dramatic turnaround. Doctors routinely recommend a healthy diet to patients with high blood glucose, but it usually only makes a marginal difference. Intermittent fasting could have a game-changing effect on the nation's health.

Fasting and cancer

My father was a lovely man but not a particularly healthy one. Overweight for much of his life, by the time he reached his 60s he had developed not only diabetes but also prostate cancer. He had an operation to remove the cancer which left him with embarrassing urinary problems. Understandably, I am not at all keen to go down that road.

My four-day fast, under Professor Valter Longo's supervision, had shown me that it was possible to dramatically cut my IGF-1 (Insulin-like Growth Factor 1) levels and by doing so, hopefully, my prostate cancer risk. I later discovered that intermittent fasting had a similar effect on my IGF-1 levels. The link between growth, fasting and cancer is worth unpacking.

The cells in our bodies are constantly multiplying, replacing dead, worn-out or damaged tissue. This is fine as long as cellular growth is under control, but sometimes a cell mutates, grows uncontrollably and turns into a cancer. Very high levels in the blood of a cellular stimulant, like IGF-1, are likely to increase the chance of this happening.

When a cancer goes rogue, the normal options are surgery, chemotherapy or radiotherapy. Surgery is used to try to remove the tumour; chemotherapy and radiotherapy are there to try and poison it. The major problem with chemotherapy and radiotherapy is that they are not selective; as well as killing tumour cells they will kill or damage surrounding healthy cells. They are particularly likely to damage rapidly dividing cells such as hair roots, which is why hair commonly falls out following therapy.

As I mentioned above, Valter Longo has shown that when we are deprived of food for even quite short periods of time, our body responds by slowing things down, going into repair and survival mode until food is once more abundant. That is true of normal cells. But cancer cells follow their own rules. They are, almost by defin-ition, not under control and will go on selfishly proliferating whatever the circumstances. This 'selfishness' creates an opportunity. If you fast just before chemotherapy, at least in theory, you create a situation where your normal cells are hibernating while the cancer cells are running amok and therefore more vulnerable.

In a paper published in 2008, Valter and his colleagues showed that fasting 'protects normal but not cancer cells against high-dose chemotherapy'.[18] They followed this with another paper in which they showed that fasting increased the efficacy of chemotherapy drugs against a variety of cancers.[19]

Again, as is so often the case, this was a study done with mice. A more recent study, which involved making dogs with advanced cancer fast for 24 hours before chemo-therapy, showed that doing so significantly reduced the risk of nausea and vomiting. Only 10% of the dogs that were fasted vomited after treatment, compared to 67%

of dogs who ate normally (http://www.ncbi.nlm.nih.gov/pubmed/24831580).

Although the research has so far largely been done with animals, the implications of Valter's work were not missed by an eagle-eyed judge called Nora Quinn, who saw a short article about it in *The LA Times*.

Nora's story

I met Nora in Los Angeles. She is a feisty woman with a terrific, dry sense of humour. Nora first noticed she had a problem when, one morning, she put her hand on her breast and felt a lump the size of a walnut under her skin. After indulging, as she put it, in the fantasy that it was a cyst, it was removed and sent to a pathologist.

'The reality of your life always comes out in pathology,' she told me. When the pathology report came back it said that she had invasive breast cancer. She had a course of radiotherapy and was about to start chemotherapy when she read about Professor Longo's work with mice.

She tried to speak to Valter, but he wouldn't advise her because none of the trials he had run, up to that point, had been done with humans. He didn't know if it was safe for someone about to undergo chemo to fast and he certainly wasn't going to encourage people like Nora to give it a go.

Undeterred, Nora did her own research and decided to

go on fasting for a seven-and-a-half-day, water-only fast to cover before, during and after chemotherapy. Having discovered how tough it can be to do even a four-day fast while fully healthy, I'm surprised she was able to go through with it, though Nora says it's not so hard and I'm just a wimp. The results were mixed: 'After the first chemo I didn't get that sick, but my hair fell out.'

So next time she didn't fast, and she was only medium sick. 'I thought it wasn't working. I thought, seven and a half days of fasting to avoid being medium sick, this is a really bad deal. I am so not doing that again.'

When it was time for her third course of chemo, she didn't fast. That, she now feels, was a mistake. 'I got sick. I don't have words for how sick I was. I was weak, felt poisoned, and I couldn't get up. I felt like I was moving through jello. It was absolutely horrible.'

The cells that line the gut, like hair root cells, grow rapidly because they need to be constantly replaced. That's one reason why chemotherapy can make people feel really ill.

By the time Nora had to undergo her fourth course of chemo she had decided once again to try fasting. This time things went much better and she made a good recovery. She is currently cancer free.

Nora is convinced she benefited from fasting but it's hard to be sure because she wasn't part of a proper medical trial. Valter and his colleagues at the University of Southern California did, however, study what happened to her and ten other patients with cancers who had also decided to put themselves on a fast.[20]

All of them reported fewer and less severe symptoms after chemotherapy and most of them, including Nora, saw improvements in their blood results. The white cells and platelets, for example, recovered more rapidly when they had chemo in a fasted state than when they did not. But why did Nora go rogue? Why didn't she fast under proper supervision?

'I decided to fast based on years of information from animal testing. I do agree that if you are going to do crazy things like I do you should have medical supervision. But how? None of my doctors would listen to me.'

Nora's self-experiment could have gone wrong, which is just one reason why such maverick behaviour is not recommended. Her experience, however, and that of the other nine cancer patients, helped inspire further studies.

For example, Professor Valter Longo and his colleagues have recently completed Phase I of a clinical trial to see if fasting around the time of chemotherapy is safe, which it seems to be. The next thing is to assess whether it makes a measurable difference. At least ten other hospitals around the world are either doing or have agreed to do clinical trials. Go to our website for the latest updates.

Fasting and chronic inflammation

Asthma

One of the other unexpected benefits of intermittent fasting is its effects on allergic diseases such as asthma and eczema. These are autoimmune diseases, the result of an overactive immune system that is mistakenly attacking the body's own cells. You might imagine that if intermittent fasting leads to new, more active white cells then this in turn could make your asthma worse. Far from it.

On our website (thefastdiet.co.uk) several people have reported seeing improvements in their asthma since going on our diet.

DB, aged 44, went on the Fast Diet and lost a stone in a month, but more unexpectedly she also saw big improvements in her lung function.

'I have changed nothing else at all, it can only be related to the Fast Diet,' DB writes. As an experiment she decided to stop doing the diet for a while.

'Guess what? My lung function tests have deteriorated significantly. Nothing else has changed. So for me that's proof enough, I am back on the diet tomorrow.'

Unfortunately there has not been a lot of scientific research looking at whether intermittent fasting is genuinely helpful for asthma. A few years ago Professor Mark Mattson, of the National Institute on Aging, with Dr James Johnson, did do a small pilot study of intermittent fasting with ten obese asthmatics (eight women and two men).[21]

The overweight asthmatics were put on an alternate day fasting diet for eight weeks. While on this diet they could eat what they wanted one day, then the following day they were asked to cut down to 20% of their normal calories.

Nine of the ten volunteers managed to stick to the diet for the two months of the trial and actually reported feeling more energetic. They lost an impressive amount of weight, an average of 8.5kg (around 17lb) but what was more surprising was that within a couple of weeks of starting intermittent fasting their asthma symptoms also improved.

Other studies have shown that people who are overweight can experience improvements in their asthma if they lose a lot of weight (at least 13% of previous body weight), but the improvements they saw in this study started long before significant weight loss.

It seems something else was going on. The likeliest explanation is that ADF led to a big drop in inflammatory markers. Certainly levels of tumour necrosis factor, a measure of chronic inflammation, fell dramatically over the course of the study. Since asthma is largely a disease of inflammation (inflamed airways make breathing harder), anything which reduces that is likely to help.

Eczema

Inflammation is also a characteristic feature of eczema (also known as dermatitis), an incredibly common skin condition. Eczema affects around 10% of people in Europe and the US. It can be mild, with occasional flare-ups when the skin becomes dry, scaly and itchy. Or it can be severe, in which case you get weeping, crusting and bleeding. My daughter had eczema when she was young and we had to battle constantly to stop her scratching. Fortunately, like many children, the eczema disappeared when she hit her teens, but there is always the risk it will return.

We have had a number of people contact us to say their eczema unexpectedly improved once they started doing the Fast Diet.

For example, B wrote to say, 'For several years I have had eight to ten mildly irritating small eczema patches on my arms and torso. Since I have been doing intermittent fasting the patches are much, much milder and a few have just disappeared.'

Tracy also wrote about the improvements she'd seen: 'The total disappearance of my eczema (used to get quite irritating recurring patches between my fingers) was one of the earliest and happiest side effects of the lifestyle for me. My skin is a million times better in general but the eczema disappearance has made this well worth doing for that reason alone.'

Unfortunately I can't find any decent studies which

have investigated the impact of intermittent fasting on eczema, but if you have eczema and decide to give it a go, do let us know how you get on.

Psoriasis

Psoriasis is an inflammatory skin condition which studies suggest may benefit from short periods of fasting. Psoriasis can look a lot like eczema. It normally consists of red or silvery, scaly patches that itch. It can appear in just a few places or cover almost the entire body.

A review article recently published in the *British Journal of Dermatology*[22] asked whether diet made any difference. Among the studies was one in which 20 patients with arthritis and various skin diseases were put on a two-week modified fast, followed by a three-week vegetarian diet. Not everyone got better, but some patients experienced an improvement. The article concluded that 'short-term fasting periods may improve severe symptoms'.

Certainly Annette, one of our followers at thefastdiet. co.uk, thinks the Fast Diet helped her psoriasis. Last year she wrote to us to say, 'I used to wake myself up scratching and sore. I started the 5:2 and within days, noticed an improvement. This has continued over the weeks to the point where I can now wear a skirt without tights, unthinkable before I started this diet.'

Again, more research is badly needed.

Intermittent fasting: my personal journey

As you've read, I started out by trying the four-day fast under Professor Valter Longo's supervision. But despite the improvements in my blood biochemistry and his obvious enthusiasm, I could not imagine doing lengthy fasts on a regular basis for the rest of my life.

Then, having met Dr Krista Varady and learnt all about ADF (Alternate Day Fasting), I decided to give that a go. After a short while, however, I realised that it was just too tough, physically, socially and psychologically. It is undoubtedly an effective way to lose weight rapidly and to get powerful changes to your biochemistry, but it was not for me.

And so I came to the idea of eating 600 calories for two days a week. It seemed a reasonable compromise and, more importantly, doable. The 5:2 Fast Diet is based on a number of different forms of intermittent fasting; it is not based on any one body of research, but is a synthesis.

Before embarking on the diet, I decided to get myself properly tested, to see what effects it would have on my body. The following are the tests I did. Most are straightforward. The blood tests are, with one exception, tests your doctor should be happy to do for you.

Get on the scales

The first and most obvious thing you will want to do is weigh yourself before embarking on this adventure. Initially, it is best to do this at the same time every day. First thing in the morning is, as I'm sure you know, when you will be at your lightest.

Ideally you should get a weighing machine that measures body-fat percentage as well as weight, since what you really want to see is body-fat levels fall. The cheaper machines are not fantastically reliable; they tend to underestimate the true figure, giving you a false sense of security. What they are quite good at doing, however, is measuring change. In other words, they might tell you when you start that you are 30% body fat when the true figure is closer to 33%. But they should be able to tell you when that number begins to fall.

Body fat

Body fat is measured as a percentage of total weight. The machines you can buy do this by a system called impedence. There's a small electric current that runs through your body and the machine measures the resistance. It does its estimation based on the fact that muscle and other tissues are better conductors of electricity than fat.

The best way to get a truly accurate figure is with a

machine called a DXA (formerly DEXA) scan. It stands for 'Dual Energy X-ray Absorptiometry'. It is relatively inexpensive and far more reliable than, say Body Mass Index. Women tend to have more body fat than men. A man with body fat of more than 25% would be considered overweight. For a woman it would be 30%.

Calculate your BMI

BMI has its critics (someone who has a lot of muscle could get a high BMI score), but it is still one of the standard ways of measuring if you are in the healthy weight zone, or not. To calculate your BMI, go to a website such as www.nhs.uk/tools/pages/healthyweightcalculator.aspx, or to thefastdiet.co.uk where you can track other indices.

Measure your stomach

BMI is useful but it may not be the best predictor of future health. In a study of over 45,000 women followed for 16 years, the waist-to-height ratio was a superior predictor of who would develop heart disease. The reason why the waist matters so much is that visceral fat, which collects inside the abdomen, is the worst sort of fat, because it causes inflammation and puts you at much higher risk of diabetes. You don't need fancy equipment to tell you if you have internal fat. All you need is a tape measure.

Male or female, your waist should be less than half your height. Most people underestimate their waist size by about two inches because they rely on trouser size. Instead, measure your waist by putting the tape measure around your belly button. Be honest. A definition of optimism is someone who steps on the scale, while holding their breath. You are fooling no one.

Blood tests

You should be able to get standard tests on the NHS.

> Fasting glucose. I chose to measure my fasting glucose because it is a really important measure of fitness, even if you are not at risk of diabetes, and a predictor of future health. Studies show that even moderately elevated levels of blood glucose are associated with increased risk of heart disease, stroke and long-term cognitive problems. Ideally I would have had my insulin sensitivity measured, but that test is complex and expensive.

Cholesterol. They measure two types of cholesterol: LDL (low-density lipoprotein) and HDL (high-density lipoprotein). Broadly speaking, LDL carries cholesterol into the wall of your arteries while HDL carries it away. It is good to have a low-ish LDL and a highish HDL. One way you can express this is as a percentage: HDL to HDL + LDL. Anything over 20% is good.

Triglycerides. These are a type of fat that is found in blood; they are one of the ways that the body stores calories. High levels are associated with increased risk of heart disease.

IGF-1. This is an expensive test and not available on the NHS. It is a measure of cell turnover and therefore of cancer risk. It may also be a marker for biological ageing. I wanted to find out the effects of 5:2 fasting on my IGF-1. I had discovered that IGF-1 levels drop dramatically in response to a four-day fast, but after a month of normal eating they bounced right back to where they had been before.

My data

These are the results of the physical measurements I took before starting the Fast Diet:

	ME	RECOMMENDED
HEIGHT	5' 11"	
WEIGHT	187lb	
BODY MASS INDEX	26.4	19–25
BODY FAT	28%	Less than 25% for men
WAIST SIZE	36"	Less than half your height
NECK SIZE	17"	Less than 16.5"

I wasn't obese, but both my BMI and my body-fat percentage told me that I was overweight. I knew from doing an MRI scan that much of my fat was collected internally, wrapping itself in thick layers around my liver and kidneys, disturbing all sorts of metabolic pathways.

Clearly, the fat wasn't all inside my abdomen. Quite a bit had collected around my neck. This meant that I was snoring. Loudly. Neck size is a powerful predictor of whether you will snore or not.[23] A neck size above 16.5" for men or 16" for women means you are in the danger zone.

	MY RESULTS in mmol/l	RECOMMENDED
DIABETES RISK: FASTING GLUCOSE	7.3	3.9–5.8
HEART DISEASE FACTORS: TRIGLYCERIDES HDL CHOLESTEROL LDL CHOLESTEROL	1.4 1.8 5.5	Less than 2.3 0.9–1.5 Up to 3.0
HEART DISEASE RISK HDL % of total	23%	20% and over
CANCER RISK Somatomedin-C (IGF-1)	28.6 nmol/l	11.3–30.9nmol/l

According to this data, my fasting glucose was worryingly high. I was a diabetic, so far only at the lower end of the range, but clearly heading towards trouble. My LDL was far too high, but I was to some extent protected by the fact that my triglycerides were low and my HDL high. This is not a good picture, though.

My IGF-1 levels were also too high, suggesting rapid turnover of cells and increased cancer risk.

After three months on the Fast Diet there were some remarkable changes.

	ME	RECOMMENDED
HEIGHT	5' 11"	
WEIGHT	168lb	
BODY MASS INDEX	24	19–25

BODY FAT	21%	Less than 25% for men
WAIST SIZE	33"	Less than half your height
NECK SIZE	16"	Less than 16.5"

I had lost about 19lb, almost one and a half stone. My BMI and body-fat percentage were now respectable. I had to go out and buy smaller belts and tighter trousers. I could fit into a dinner jacket I hadn't worn for ten years. I had also stopped snoring, which delighted my wife and quite possibly the neighbours. Even better, my blood indicators had improved in a spectacular fashion.

	MY RESULTS in mmol/l	RECOMMENDED
DIABETES RISK: FASTING GLUCOSE	5.0	3.9–5.8
HEART DISEASE FACTORS: TRIGLYCERIDES HDL CHOLESTEROL LDL CHOLESTEROL	0.6 2.1 3.6	Less than 2.3 0.9–1.5 Up to 3.0
HEART DISEASE RISK HDL % of total	37%	20% and over
CANCER RISK Somatomedin-C (IGF-1)	15.9nmol/l	11.3–30.9nmol/l

My wife Clare, who is a doctor, was astonished. She regularly sees overweight patients with blood chemistry like mine had been and she said that none of the advice she gives has anything like the same effect.

For me, the particularly pleasing changes were in my fasting glucose levels and the huge drop in my IGF-1 levels, which matched the changes I had seen after doing a four-day fast.

Clare, however, felt I was losing weight too fast, that I should consolidate for a while. So I decided to go on a 6:1 maintenance programme, fasting just one day a week.

What has happened over the last two years is that my weight has stayed broadly around 12 stone and my bloods remain in good shape. There are times, around the holiday season, when my weight creeps up, in which case I either go back to 5:2 or have a few days where I just skip lunch. These days I also do more exercise.

Adding exercise

It won't surprise you to learn that doing exercise, in conjunction with intermittent fasting, will help you lose more weight (fat, in particular), and it will certainly improve your general fitness, strength and health – which, of course, is the overarching goal.

Which exercise is best?

The best exercise is the one you like best, the one you'll actually do. Even a small amount can really make a difference – studies show that a few short bouts of general activity throughout the day can promote cardiovascular and respiratory health, lower your risk of diabetes and improve your longevity.

You can do it almost any way you want: running, walking, swimming or by undertaking some vigorous housework. I find on a Fast Day that a brisk walk or a quick run up and down the stairs helps curb hunger pangs.

The benefits of exercise plus intermittent fasting

Dr Krista Varady recently did a study which compared the effectiveness of intermittent fasting with and without an exercise regime.[24]

In this study she got 64 overweight volunteers and randomly allocated them to four groups. One group did ADF. Another did ADF plus three sessions of 40 minutes moderate intensity exercise a week, on an exercise bike or an elliptical trainer. The third group just did this exercise, and the fourth group acted as a control.

The volunteers did this for 12 weeks and at the end of the trial the ADF-plus-exercise group were the clear winners. They had lost an average of 6kg (13lb), compared to 3kg for the ADF group and just 1kg for those who only did the exercise. The ADF-plus-exercise group also saw the biggest improvements in things like their blood cholesterol score.

To get the benefit, the volunteers in this study were doing 120 minutes of moderate intensity exercise a week, slightly less that the recommended levels of 150 minutes a week.

The problem is, despite the fact we know it's good for us, all too few of us are prepared to put aside that much time. That has certainly been my excuse.

So a while ago I began looking into a radically different approach to exercise called HIT, High Intensity Training. The idea is you can get many of the more important benefits of exercise from just a few minutes of HIT a week.

Jamie Timmons, Professor of Precision Medicine at King's College, London, has spent many years researching the benefits HIT.

When we first met he assured me that a few minutes of HIT a week had been shown to improve the body's ability to cope with sugar surges (metabolic fitness), and how good the heart and lungs are at getting oxygen into the body (aerobic fitness). These two measures are great predictors of future health.

Intrigued, I had blood taken and went through some baseline tests to assess my starting point, fitness-wise. Then I began to do HIT.

The version I chose was very simple. I got on an exercise bike, warmed up by doing gentle cycling for a couple of minutes, then started to pick up the pace. At the same time I increased the resistance on the bike, pushing the dial to one of the highest levels, so I was going flat-out against almost maximum resistance for 20 seconds.

I then cycled gently for a couple of minutes, long enough to catch my breath, then did another 20 seconds at full throttle. Another couple of minutes' gentle cycling, then a final 20 seconds going hell for leather. And that was it.

I did three sessions of HIT a week for four weeks (12 minutes of intense exercise in total) and then went back to the lab to be retested.

The main surprise was the effect it had on my insulin sensitivity. After 12 minutes of intense exercise my insulin sensitivity had improved by a remarkable 24%, something you would be unlikely to see after many hours of conventional exercise. It was extremely satisfying.

I also found that doing HIT improved my mood and helped control my appetite.

Combining 5:2 with HIT

There have been studies looking at intermittent fasting, and studies looking at HIT, but until recently no one had evaluated a programme combining the two.

So I was delighted when I was contacted by Dr Ray Power, who is based in Dublin, where he runs a wellness clinic, and who wanted to test it.

Ray was once a fit young rugby player. But then, like many middle-aged men, he allowed his weight to creep up until one day he stepped on the scales and realised that he weighed over 97kg.

'I was exercising three times per week and being a sensible Jim,' he said, 'but none of that made any difference. I couldn't shift the weight. I knew it was unhealthy; I had to grasp the nettle, do something.'

I put him in touch with Professor Jamie Timmons, and with his help Ray put together a 12-week programme which he calls iFast. He also decided, following the long traditions of medical self-experimentation, that he should start by testing out the programme on himself. 'I was apprehensive,' he said, 'not of the exercise but of the fasting – I had never done a diet before in my life.'

Before he started, he had a DXA scan done (important if you want to accurately measure fat loss) and a range of blood tests.

Ray stuck rigorously to 600 calories twice a week, but didn't significantly change his lifestyle on the other five days. He also did three bursts of HIT a week. 'It works for my Irish psyche,' he told me, 'I am an all-or-nothing kind of bloke and the fact that I can take the foot off the pedal for a couple of days and give it my normal rattle the rest of the time sits perfectly with my personality.'

Twelve weeks later he got himself retested and the results were impressive.

Ray lost over 16lb (7.5kg), all of it fat. He also lost three inches from his waist and his cholesterol levels improved significantly. His IGF-1 is now very low and he says, 'I feel fantastic; it definitely has given me a spring in my stride.'

The iFast dieters

Having tested it on himself, Ray then put 20 volunteers through a similar programme. They all had DXA scans before and after, as well as blood tests.

On average they lost slightly over 4.6kg (10lb), with one dieter losing an impressive 12.6kg.

What was encouraging was that almost all of the weight the dieters lost was fat; there was almost no loss of muscle. This is important because, as well as making you look toned, muscle is metabolically active; it keeps burning calories even when you are asleep. With some diets up to 30% of weight loss can be muscle, and with crash diets it can be 40% or higher.

Another encouraging finding was that the dieters, just like Ray, had lost an average of over three inches around the waist. Fat that settles around your gut is the most harmful, increasing your risk of heart disease and diabetes. There were also significant improvements in cholesterol, IGF-1 and fasting insulin levels (reducing their risk of diabetes and some cancers) – all very good reasons to give a combination of the 5:2 diet and HIT a go.

Strength training

Good though cycling, running or walking are for your heart and lungs, it is also important that you add some weight or resistance training, to help your body build more lean muscle and maintain bone density.

These days I combine HIT, three times a week, with a very simple strength and flexibility regime, also about three times a week. The combination, which takes less than 30 minutes a week, has led to some impressive biceps and the beginnings of a six-pack. If you want to find out more, I have written a book with sports journalist Peta Bee called *Fast Exercise*. A free app, Fast Exercise, is also available to download from the App Store.

So how can you achieve so much change in so little time? Part of the explanation is that HIT makes your muscles produce new and more efficient mitochondria, the tiny power plants in your cells that convert the food you eat into the energy you burn. The more mitochondria you have, the more power they produce and the more fat and sugar they consume.

Like fasting, HIT is a shock to the system and the stress caused by HIT leads to the release of large amounts of catecholamines – hormones like adrenaline and noradrenaline – which target fat cells, particularly those in the abdomen.

Not everyone is going to enjoy pushing themselves really hard, even if it is only for 20 seconds. Yet in trials most people say they prefer it to conventional exercise, not least because it is over so quickly. And the good news is that it seems to be safe to do even if you are older or less fit.

A recent study from Abertay University in Scotland reported on a group of unfit volunteers aged between 65 and 75 who were asked to do a few very short sessions (10 bursts of 6 seconds) of high intensity pedalling on an exercise bike.[25] Done twice a week, this was enough to produce some impressive changes. As the scientist behind the experiment, Dr John Babraj, explained, 'What we found with this study – which involves doing just one minute of exercise twice a week – is that it not only improved the participants' physical health and ability to do things, but also their perceptions of their own ability to engage in physical activity.'

Clearly people who are older need to take things more gently when they start, but there is a persistent and over-stated fear that exercise in later life will lead to heart attacks and strokes. The reverse is true.

So, what is the best way to go about an intermittent fast?

Let's recap on what we've learnt. The reason for intermittent fasting – briefly but severely restricting the amount of calories you consume – is that by doing so you are hoping to 'fool' your body into thinking it is in a potential famine situation and that it needs to switch from go-go mode to maintenance mode.

The reason our bodies respond to fasting in this way is that we evolved at a time when feast and famine were the norm. Our bodies are designed to respond to stresses and shocks; it makes them healthier, tougher. The scientific term is hormesis – that which does not kill you makes you stronger. The benefits of fasting include:

- Weight loss

- A reduction in IGF-1, which means that you are reducing your risk of a number of age-related diseases, such as cancer

- The switching-on of countless repair genes in response to this stressor

- A rest for your pancreas, which will boost the effectiveness of the insulin it produces in response to elevated blood glucose. Increased insulin sensitivity will reduce your risk of obesity, diabetes, heart disease and cognitive decline

- An overall enhancement in your mood and sense of wellbeing. This may be a consequence of your brain producing increased levels of neurotrophic factor,

which will hopefully make you more cheerful, which
in turn should make fasting more doable

So much for the science. In the next chapter Mimi discusses what to eat and how to go about starting life as an intermittent faster. How do you put the theory into practice?

THE FAST DIET IN PRACTICE

There are, as we've seen, good clinical reasons to start intermittent fasting. Some, such as its positive effect on blood markers, should be immediately apparent; others will become manifest over time – a cognitive boost, a self-repairing physiology, a greater chance of a longer life. But perhaps the most compelling argument for many is the promise of swift and sustained weight loss, while still eating the foods you enjoy, most of the time. You may view this as incidental to the plan's other marked health benefits. Or it may be your primary objective. The fact is you will gain both. Weight loss and better health, two sides of the same page.

Michael's experience, as described in the previous chapter, will have given you an idea of what to expect. In this chapter I will reveal more detail – explaining how to start, how it will feel, how to keep going and how the central tenets of the Fast Diet can slip easily into the rhythm of your everyday life.

Now, it's over to you.

What do 500-600 calories look like?

Cutting calories to a quarter of your usual daily intake is a significant commitment, so don't be surprised if your first Fast Day feels like a tough gig. As you progress, the fasts will become second nature and the initial sense of deprivation will diminish, particularly if you remain aware that tomorrow is another day – another day, in fact, when you can eat normally again.

Still, however you cut it, 500 or 600 calories is no picnic; it's not even half a picnic. A large café latte can clock in at over 300 calories, more if you insist on cream, while your usual lunchtime sandwich might easily consume your entire allowance in one huge bite. So be smart. Spend your calories wisely – the menu plans and recipes on pages 165-216 will be useful – but it's also worth having a clear idea of favourite Fast Day foods that work for you. Remember to embrace variety: differing textures, punchy flavours, colour and crunch. Together, these things will keep your mouth entertained and stop it frowning at the hardship of it all.

When to fast

Animal studies, human studies, research, experiment: as demonstrated in the previous chapter, evidence for the value of fasting is strong. But what happens when you step out of the laboratory and into real life? When and what you eat during your 'fast' is critical to the diet's success. So what's the optimal pattern?

Michael tried several different fasting regimes; the one he settled on as the most sustainable for him is a fast on two non-consecutive days each week, allowing 600 calories a day, split between breakfast and dinner. For obvious reasons, he named this pattern the 5:2 diet – five days off, two days on, which means that the majority of your time is spent gloriously free from calorie-counting. On a Fast Day, he'll normally have breakfast with the family at around 7.30am and then aim to have dinner with them at 7.30pm, with nothing eaten in between. That way, he gets two 12-hour fasts in a day, and a happy family at the end of it.

The menu suggestions on pages 169-91 are based on this pattern as it is, in his experience, the most straightforward intermittent fasting method.

As will become clear later in this chapter, I found that a slightly different pattern works for me. Sticking to the Fast Diet's central tenet, I eat 500 calories – but as two meals with an occasional snack (an apple, some carrot sticks) in between, simply because the vast plain between breakfast and supper feels too great, too empty for comfort. There is evidence, from trials conducted by Dr Michelle Harvie[26] and others, that this approach will help you lose weight, reduce your risk of breast cancer and increase insulin sensitivity.

Which approach is better? At this point, given that the science of intermittent fasting is still in its early days, we don't know. On purely theoretical grounds, a longer period without food (Michael's approach) might be expected to produce better results. It takes, for example, about 12 hours without food before your body switches into proper fat-burning mode. Valter Longo thinks that longer periods are better. Fasting or not, he almost always skips lunch.

Professor Mark Mattson at the National Institute on Aging says that by eating your calories as a single meal you might get a modestly greater ketogenic ('fat-burning') effect, compared to three very small meals spread through the day. But he also thinks we shouldn't get too hung up about it. 'Regardless of whether the 600 calories are consumed as one meal or two or three smaller meals, you will get major health benefits.'

As far as we are aware there have, as yet, been no studies which attempt to compare the health benefits of either eating all the calories in one go or splitting them into two meals and including the odd snack. When we know more we will update you.

In the meantime, it is clear from the many thousands who have tried it that as long as you stick to the Fast Diet you will enjoy that crucial combination of weight loss, health benefits and cheerful compliance.

Some people who don't feel hungry at breakfast would

rather eat later in the day. That's fine. One of the key researchers in this field often starts her day with a late breakfast at around 11am and finishes with supper at 7pm. Based on the mouse study cited on page 34, it may even be a better approach.

It is, however, only better if you actually do it, and a delayed breakfast may not suit some lifestyles, diaries or bodies. So go with a timetable that suits you. Some fasters will appreciate the convenience and simplicity of a single 500- or 600-calorie meal, allowing them to ignore food entirely for most of the day. Whatever you choose, it must be your plan, your life. Do it with gusto, but be prepared to experiment, within the limits set out by the plan.

What to eat

It may seem curious to talk about what to eat when you are fasting. But the Fast Diet is a modified programme, allowing 500 calories for a woman and 600 for a man on any given Fast Day, making the regime relatively comfortable and, above all, sustainable over the long term. So, yes, you do get to eat on a Fast Day. But it matters what you choose.

There are two general principles that should govern what you eat and what you avoid on a Fast Day. Your aim is to have food that makes you feel satisfied, but stays firmly within the 500/600-calorie allowance – and the best options to achieve this are meals that include:

- Foods with a low Glycaemic Index (GI)

- Some protein

There have been several studies demonstrating that individuals who eat a diet higher in protein feel fuller for longer (indeed the main reason why people lose weight on diets like Atkins is that they eat less).[27] The trouble with really high-protein diets, however, is that people tend to get bored with the food restrictions and give up. There is also evidence that high-protein diets are associated with higher levels of chronic inflammation and IGF-1, which in turn are associated with increased risk of heart disease and cancer.[28]

So the Fast Diet does not recommend boycotting carbs entirely, nor living permanently on a high-protein diet. However, on a Fast Day, the combination of proteins and foods with a low GI will be helpful weapons in keeping hunger at bay.

Understanding the Glycaemic Index

In earlier chapters, we discovered the importance of blood sugar and insulin. High levels of insulin brought about by high levels of blood sugar will encourage your body to store fat and increase your cancer risk. Another reason not to eat foods that make your blood sugar levels surge, particularly on your Fast Days, is that when your blood sugar crashes, as it inevitably will, you will start feeling very hungry indeed.

Carbohydrates have the biggest impact on blood sugars, but not all carbs are equal. As habitual dieters will know, one way to discover which carbs cause a big spike and which don't is to look at their GI. Each food gets a score out of 100, with a low score meaning that the particular food does not tend to cause a rapid rise in blood glucose. These are the ones you want.

The size of the sugar spike depends both on the food itself, and on how much of it you eat. For example, we tend to eat a lot more potatoes in one sitting than kiwi fruit. So there's also a measure called GL, the Glycaemic Load:

$$\frac{GI \times \text{grammes of carbohydrate}}{100}$$

This makes some pretty heroic assumptions about the amount of a particular food you are likely to eat as a portion, but at least it is a guide.

The reason GI and GL are interesting is not just that they are strongly predictive of future health (people on a low-GL diet have less risk of diabetes, heart disease and various cancers), but that there are so many surprises. Who would have imagined that eating a baked potato would have as big an impact on your blood glucose as eating a tablespoon of sugar?

Broadly speaking a GI over 50 or a GL over 20 is not good, and the lower both figures are the better. It is worth restating that GI and GL are measures that relate to carbs. GI is not relevant to protein and fats, which is why none of the foods listed have a significant protein or fat content. As an example, let's take a quick look at breakfast:

BREAKFAST	GI	GL
PORRIDGE	50	10
MUESLI	50	10
BAGUETTE	95	15
CROISSANT	67	17
CORNFLAKES	80	20

You can see why, if you are having a carb breakfast, porridge and muesli are better options than cornflakes or a croissant. And what are you going to put on your muesli?

	GI	GL
MILK	27	3
SOY MILK	44	8

The relatively high GI and GL of soy milk is just one reason to stick with dairy.

What about protein?

We certainly don't recommend eating protein to the exclusion of all else on a Fast Day, but you do require an adequate quantity, for muscle health, cell maintenance, endocrinal regulation, immunity and energy. Protein is satiating too, so it's well worth including it in your calorie quota. It may sound confusing that we recommend protein on your Fast Day, while elsewhere Michael suggests that too much protein is not good for you. The answer is that while we recommend eating a higher *percentage* of your diet as protein on a Fast Day, since you are eating significantly fewer calories overall, you are actually consuming relatively modest amounts of protein.

While Valter Longo recommends 0.8g of protein per kg of body weight per day – which would give a 12-stone man around 60g, and a nine-stone woman around 45g – perhaps the simplest method is to stick to recommended governmental guidelines, which allow for a (quite generous) 50g per day.

Go for 'good protein'. Steamed white fish, for example, is low in saturated fats and rich in minerals. Choose skinless chicken over red meat; try low-fat dairy products over endless lattes; include prawns, tuna, tofu and other plant proteins. Nuts, seeds, pulses and legumes are full of fibre and act as bulking agents on a hungry day. Nuts – though high in calories (depending, of course, on how many you eat) – are generally low GI and brilliantly satiating. They are fatty too, so you might imagine they are 'bad for you', yet the evidence is that nut consumers have lower rates of heart disease and diabetes than nut abstainers.[29]

Eggs, meanwhile, are low in saturated fat and full of nutritional value; they won't adversely affect your cholesterol levels and they score around 80 calories each (that's for a medium egg). What's more, research suggests that individuals who consume egg protein for breakfast are more likely to feel full during the day than those whose breakfasts contain wheat protein.[30] So an egg-based breakfast on a Fast Day makes perfect sense. Two eggs plus a 50g serving of smoked salmon, for example, clocks in at a sensible 250 calories. Poaching or boiling an egg avoids the addition of careless calories. For more suggestions about foods to keep you full on a Fast Day, and the benefits certain choices will bring, turn to page 135.

How to fit fasting into your life

When to start?

If you do not have an underlying medical condition, and if you are not an individual for whom fasting is proscribed (see pages 154-55), then there really is no time like the present. Ask yourself: if not now, when? You may prefer to await a doctor's advice. You may choose to prepare yourself, talk yourself down from a lifelong habit of overeating, clear out the fridge, eat the last cookie in the jar, have a scratch (there are plenty of tips for preparation in the pages ahead). Or you may want to get on with it and start to see visible progress within a couple of weeks. Do, however, begin on a day when you feel strong, purposeful, calm and committed. Do tell friends and family that you're starting the Fast Diet: once you make a public commitment, you are much more likely to stick with it. Avoid high days, holidays and days when you're booked in for a three-course lunch complete with bread basket, cheese board and four types of dessert.

Recognise, too, that a busy day will help your fast time fly, while a duvet day generally crawls by like honey off a spoon. Once you've deliberated and designated a day to debut, get your mind in gear. Record your details – weight, BMI, waist, target weight – before you start and note your progress in a diary, knowing that dieters who keep an honest account of what they eat and drink are more likely to lose the pounds and keep them off. Then… take a deep breath and relax. Better yet, shrug. It's no big deal, just a brief break from eating: you have nothing to lose but weight.

How tough will it be?

If it has been a while since you have experienced hunger, even the slightest hint, you'll probably find that eating no more than 500 or 600 calories in a day is a mild challenge, at least initially. Intermittent fasters do report that the process becomes significantly easier with time, particularly as they witness results in the mirror and on the scales. Though your first Fast Day may well be your most challenging, it's equally possible that it will speed by, buoyed along by the novelty of the process; a Fast Day on a wet Wednesday in week three may feel more of a slog.

Your mission is to complete it, knowing that, although you are saying no to chocolate today, you will be eating normally tomorrow. That is the joy of the Fast Diet and what makes it so different from other weight-loss plans.

How to win the hunger games

There is no reason to be alarmed by benign, occasional, short-term hunger. Given base-level good health, you will not perish. You won't collapse in a heap and need to be rescued by the cat. Your body is designed to go without food for longish periods, even if it has lost the skill through years of grazing, picking and snacking. Research has found that modern humans tend to mistake a whole range of emotions for hunger.[31] We eat when we're bored, when we're thirsty, when we're around food (when aren't we?), when we're in company or simply when the clock happens to tell us it's time for food. Most of us eat, too, just because it feels good.

This 'hedonic eating' can readily overcome the body's natural satiety signals: you'll recognise it if you eat for reasons other than hunger. The kicker might be social (shared lunches, communal eating, everyone at the table agreeing to order pudding); it may be environmental (scheduled mealtimes which persuade you that you're hungry even when you're not, the arrival of bread at the beginning of a meal), or emotional (comfort eating, the popcorn that makes a movie more of a treat, the tub of ice cream demolished when you're feeling blue). While you should try to resist hedonic eating on a Fast Day, you can bask in the knowledge that, if you please, you can give in to a little temptation the following day.

There's no need to panic about any of this. Simply note that the human brain is adept at persuading us that we're hungry in almost all situations: when faced with feelings of deprivation or withdrawal or disappointment; when angry, sad, happy, neutral; when subject to advertising, social imperatives, sensory stimulation, reward, habit, the smell of freshly brewed coffee or baking bread or bacon cooking in a café up the road. Recognise now that these are often learnt reactions to external cues, most of them designed to part you from your cash. On a Fast Day, if you are still processing your last meal, it's highly unlikely that what you are experiencing is true hunger ('total transit time', should you be interested in such things, can take up to two days, depending on your gender, your metabolism and what you've eaten).

While hunger pangs can be aggressive and disagreeable, in practice, they are more fluid and controllable than you might think. You're unlikely to be troubled at all by hunger until well into a Fast Day. What's more, a pang will pass. Fasters report that the feeling of perceived hunger comes in waves, not in an ever-growing wall of gnawing belly noise. It's a symphony of differentiated movements, not a steady, fearful crescendo. Treat a tummy rumble as a good sign, a healthy messenger.

Remember, too, that hunger does not build over a 24-hour period, so don't feel trapped in the feeling at any given moment. Wait a while. You have absolute power to conquer feelings of hunger, simply by steering your mind, riding the wave, choosing to do something else – take a walk, phone a friend, drink tea, go for a run, take a shower... After a few weeks' practising intermittent fasting, people generally report that their sense of hunger is diminished.

The main struggle with doing the Fast Diet or any form of fasting is the first few weeks while your body and mind adjust to new habits, new ways of eating. The good news is that most people find they soon adapt. In fact many people have contacted us to say that it is unexpectedly easy.

The important thing is to have a strategy that suits you. Try to decipher your hunger. Are you really hungry? Or are you overriding your brain's satiety message? Even posing the question can be enough to still the urge. There are practical ways to circumvent the feeling too: the real trick is to eat foods that keep you feeling fuller longer. This means some protein. This means slow-burn, low-GI fuel. This means bulk from plants.

Compliance and sustainability: finding a sensible eating pattern that works for you

Most diets don't work. You know that already. Indeed, when a team of psychologists at UCLA conducted an analysis of 31 long-term diet trials back in 2007, they concluded that 'several studies indicate that dieting is a consistent predictor of future weight gain... We asked what evidence there is that dieting works in the long term, and found that the evidence shows the opposite.' Their analysis found that, while slimmers on conventional diets do lose pounds in the early months, the vast majority return to their original weight within five years, while 'at least a third end up heavier than when they embarked on the project'.[32] The standard approach clearly doesn't work.

In order to be effective, then, any method must be rational, sustainable, flexible and feasible for the long haul. Adherence, not weight loss per se, is the key, so your goals must be realistic and the programme practical. It must fit into your life as it is, not the life of your dreams. It needs to go on holiday with you, it needs to visit friends, get you through a boring (or challenging) day at the office and cope with Christmas. To work at all, any weight-loss strategy has to be tolerable, organic and innate, not some spurious add-on that makes you feel awkward and self-conscious, the dietary equivalent of uncomfortable shoes.

While the long-term experience of intermittent fasters is still under investigation, people who have tried it comment on how easily it fits into everyday life. They still get variety from food (anyone who's ever tried to lose weight on 'only' grapefruit or cabbage soup will know how vital this is). They still get rewards from food. They still get a life. There is no drama, no desperate dieting, no self-flagellation. No sweat.

Tomorrow is another day: the Fast Diet's USP

Perhaps the most reassuring, and game-changing, part of the Fast Diet is that it doesn't last for ever. Unlike deprivation diets that have failed you before, on this plan, tomorrow will always be different. Easier. There may be pancakes for breakfast, or lunch with friends, wine with supper, apple pie with cream.

This On/Off switch is critical. It means that, on a Fast Day, though you're eating a quarter of your normal calorie intake, tomorrow you can eat as usual. There's boundless psychological comfort in the fact that your fasting will only ever be a short stay, a brief break from food.

When you're not fasting, ignore fasting – it doesn't

own you, it doesn't define you. You're not even doing it most of the time. Unlike full-time fad diets, you'll still get pleasure from food, you'll still have treats, you'll engage in the regular, routine, food-related events of your normal life. There are no special shakes, bars, rules, points, affectations or idiosyncrasies. No saying 'no' all the time.

For this reason, you won't feel serially deprived – which, as anyone who has embarked on the grinding chore of long-term, every-day dieting, the kind that makes you want to commit hara-kiri right there on the kitchen floor every time you open the fridge door, is precisely why conventional diet plans fail.

The key, then, is to recognise, through patience and the exercise of will, that you can make it through a Fast Day. Bear in mind that fasting subjects regularly report that the food with which they 'break their fast' tastes glorious. Flavours sing. Mouthfuls dance. If you've ever felt a lazy disregard for the food you consume without thinking, then things are about to change. There's nothing like a bit of delayed gratification to make things taste good.

Flexibility: your key to success

Your body is not my body. Mine is not yours. So it's worth carving out your plan according to your needs, the shape of your day, your family, your commitments, your preferences. We none of us live cookie-cutter lives, and no single diet plan fits all. Everyone has quirks and qualifiers. That's why there are no absolute commandments here, just suggestions. You may choose to fast in a particular way, on a particular day. You may like to eat once, or twice, first thing or last. You may like beetroot or fennel or blueberries.

Some individuals prefer to be told exactly what to eat and when; others like a more informal approach. That's fine. It's enough to simply stick to the basic method – 500 or 600 calories a day, with as long a window without food as possible, twice a week – and you'll gain the plan's multiple benefits. In time, there's little need for assiduous calorie counting; you'll know what a Fast Day means and how to make it suit you. You can, however, stack the odds in your favour... by changing your mind.

Mind and motivation: how to master habit, temptation and willpower

Since we first published *The Fast Diet* back in 2012, one of the topics that has regularly come up in the chat rooms and on our website – and in the street or in the coffee queue – is how to deal with ingrained habits around food. Fasting, even for relatively short periods, even with calories coming in, quite obviously requires not only self-motivation, but a generous degree of self-control.

On average, we make 227 food-related decisions every

day (most people, when questioned, wildly underestimate the number and guess that it's about 14).[33] That's plenty of choice, and plenty of opportunities to collapse into the embrace of the nearest gingerbread man. Over the last two years, we've compiled some strategies to help you arm yourself against temptation. The basic message is to notice *in advance* the traps and the tripwires to come. These will be personal to you – your very own map of habits and routines that may frustrate a Fast Day. A few tips should help you navigate the terrain ahead.

- *Know your triggers.* When you experience a compulsion to eat too much, or to break a fast, it's time to face it head on. You are a rational being and you are making a specific, time-sensitive decision to eat that sandwich or pour that glass of wine. You really do have the power to choose, at each incremental, individual moment. Once you appreciate this power, it is possible to overcome the cognitive bias that leads to impulsive snacking and compulsive eating – certainly for long enough to get you through a Fast Day. Recognise – before it happens – when your self-control is likely to dissolve. Try to install a behaviour – not for ever, just for that precise moment – which alters your established route. This is called 'deliberate practice'; it takes grit, determination and a certain amount of self-awareness. If, for instance, you're always ravenous when you get home from work on a

Fast Day, make sure there's an apple stashed in your bag to eat en route (and include it in your calorie count for that day). Have business lunches in the office or in a park, not in a restaurant where they serve the world's best tiramisu. If you're prone to a late-night forage in the fridge, run a bath instead

- *Understand that temptation, when it comes, is fleeting.* Prepare to distract yourself, if only for five minutes – count backwards, concentrate on your breathing, sing, nip upstairs to make the bed, fetch a glass of water, stroll across the office to speak to a friend. Small actions? Yes, but powerful enough for that particular and distinct moment of craving to pass

- *Employ the 'proximity principle' and put temptation out of reach.* As one study (using Hershey's Kisses) showed, having food conveniently close at hand makes you eat a great deal more of it.[34] On a Fast Day, don't give yourself the choice of whether to eat the biscuits or not; hide the biscuits. Better yet, don't buy the biscuits. Buy more fresh vegetables and have them handy instead

- *Ensure that your goal outweighs your temptation.* This may seem obvious (otherwise, you'd never get going). But you need reminding, at the very instant of seduction, that you're fasting for very good reasons:

for weight loss, better health, longer life. Perhaps try site-specific aversion therapy. If necessary, tape a picture of yourself – the selfie you'd never post on Facebook, the holiday snap that made you embark on the Fast Diet in the first place – to the fridge door

- *Exercise willpower.* I mean really 'exercise' it. In her book *The Willpower Instinct*, Stanford psychologist Kelly McGonigal suggests that self-control shouldn't be seen as a virtue, but as a muscle: it gets tired from use, but regular exercise makes it stronger. This is great news: it means (as we know from experience on the Fast Diet) that the going gets easier if we persevere

The Maintenance Model

Once you've reached your target weight, or just a shade below (allowing room for manoeuvre and a generous slice of birthday cake), you may consider adopting the Maintenance Model. This is an adjustment to fasting on just one day each week – going from 5:2 to 6:1 – in order to remain in a holding pattern at your desired weight, but still reap the benefits of occasional fasting.

Naturally, one day a week may offer fewer health benefits than two in the long run; but it does fit neatly into a life, particularly if you are not intent on achieving any further weight loss.

Equally, if the beach beckons or there's a wedding in the diary or you've woken up on Boxing Day haunted by that fourth roast potato, step it up again. You're in charge.

What to expect

The first thing you can expect from adopting the Fast Diet, of course, is to lose weight: some weeks more, some weeks less; some weeks finding yourself stuck at a disappointing plateau, other weeks making swifter progress. As a basic guide, you might anticipate a loss of around one to two pounds a week. This will not, of course, be all fat. Some will be water, and the digested food in your system. You should, however, lose around ten pounds of fat over a ten-week period, which beats a typical low-calorie diet. Crucially, you can expect to maintain your weight loss over time.

More important than what you'll lose, though, is what you're set to gain…

How your anatomy will change

Over a period of weeks, you can expect your BMI, your levels of body fat and your waist measurement to gradually fall. Your cholesterol and triglyceride levels may improve. This is the path to greater health and extended life. You are already dodging your unwritten future. Right now, though, the palpable changes will start to show up in the mirror as your body becomes leaner and lighter.

As the weeks progress, you'll find that intermittent fasting has potent secondary effects too. Alongside the obvious weight loss and the health benefits stored up for the future, there are more subtle consequences, perks and bonuses that can come into play.

How your appetite will change

Expect your food preferences to adapt; pretty soon, you'll start to choose healthy foods by default rather than by design. You will begin to understand hunger, to negotiate and manage it, knowing how it feels to be properly hungry; you'll also recognise the sensation of being pleasantly full, not groaning like an immovable sofa. Satiated, not stuffed. The upshot? No more 'food hangovers', improved digestion, more bounce.

After six months of intermittent fasting, interesting things should happen to your eating habits. You may find that you eat half the meat you once did – not as a conscious move, but as a natural one born of what you desire rather than what you decide or believe. You're likely to consume more veg. Many intermittent fasters instinctively retreat from bread (and, by association, butter), while stodgy 'comfort' foods seem less appealing and refined sugars aren't nearly as tempting as they once were.

Of course, you don't need to dwell actively on any of this. It will happen anyway. If you are like me, then one day soon, you'll arrive at a place where you say no to the cheesecake because you don't fancy it, not because you are denying yourself a treat.

This is the baseline power of intermittent fasting: it encourages you to recheck your diet. And that's your long-haul ticket to health.

How your attitude will change

So, yes, you'll start to lose bad habits around food. But if you continue to fast – and eat – with awareness, all kinds of other changes should occur, some of them unlikely and unexpected.

You may, for instance, discover that you've been suffering from 'portion distortion' for years, thinking that the food piled on your plate is the quantity you really need and want. With time, you'll probably discover that you've been overdoing it. Muffins will start to look vast as they sit, fat and moist, under glass domes in coffee shops. A maxi bag of crisps becomes a monstrous prospect. You may go from Venti to Grande to wanting only half a cup, no sugar, no cream.

Soon, you'll come to recognise the truth about how

you've been eating and the wordless fibs you've told your-self for years. This is as much a part of the recalibrating process as anything else; you've changed your mind. Occasional fasting will train you in the art of 'restrained eating'; in the last instance, this is the goal. It's all part of the long game of behavioural change that means that the Fast Diet will ultimately become neither a fast, nor a diet, but a way of life.

After a while, you'll have cultivated a new approach to eating – thoughtful, rational, responsible – without even knowing you're doing it.

Intermittent fasters also report a boost in their energy, together with an amplified sense of emotional wellbeing. Some talk of a 'glow' – the result, perhaps, of winning the battle for self-control, or of the smaller clothes and the compliments, or of something going on at a meta-bolic level that governs our moods. We may not yet know precisely why, but whatever it is, it feels good. Far better than cake. As one online devotee says, 'Overall, fasting just seems right. It's like a reset button for your entire body.'[35]

More subtly still, many fasters acknowledge a sense of relief as their Fast Days no longer revolve around food. Embrace it. There's a certain liberty here, if you allow it to materialise. You may find, as we have, that you start to look forward to your fasts: a time to regroup and give feeding a rest.

The Fast Diet in reality:
tales, tips and troubleshooting

How men fast: Michael's experience

A lot of men have contacted me over the last two years to let me know how much weight they have lost and also to say how surprised and delighted they are that intermittent fasting turns out to be so easy. They like its simplicity, the fact that you don't have to give things up or try to remember complicated recipes. I also think they rather like the challenge.

One of the things that men seem to like particularly about fasting is that they can fit it into their lives with minimal hassle. It doesn't stop them working, travelling, socialising or exercising. In fact, some find it fuels performance (see page 151 for more on fasting and exercise).

In one Belgian study, men asked to eat a high-fat diet and exercise before breakfast on an empty stomach put on far less weight than a similar group of men on an identical diet who exercised after breakfast.[36] This study lends support to the claim that exercising in a fasted state makes the body burn a greater percentage of fat for fuel. At least it does if you are a man.

For me, a Fast Day now follows a familiar routine. I start with a protein-rich breakfast, normally scrambled eggs or kippers. I drink several cups of black coffee and tea during the day, work happily through lunch and rarely feel any hunger pangs until well into the late afternoon. When they happen, I simply ignore them or go for a brief stroll until they pass.

In the evening I have a bit of meat or fish and piles of steamed vegetables. Having abstained since breakfast I find them particularly delicious.

I never have problems getting to sleep and most times wake up the next morning feeling no more peckish than normal.

How women fast: Mimi's experience

While most men I know respond well to numbers and targets (with associated gadgets if at all possible), I've found that women tend to take a more holistic approach to fasting. As with much in life, we like to examine how it feels, knowing that our bodies are unique and will respond to any given stimulation in their own sweet way. We respond to shared stories and the support of friends. And, sometimes, we need a snack.

Personally, for instance, I like to consume my Fast Day calories in two lots, one early, one late, bookending the day with my allowance and aiming for a longish gap in between to maximise the prospect of health gains and weight loss. But I do sometimes need a little something to keep me going in between. A Fast Day breakfast is usually a low-sugar muesli, perhaps including some fresh strawberries and almonds, with semi-skimmed milk; there'll be an apple 'for lunch' – hardly a feast, I know, but just enough to make a difference to the day. Then, supper at 7-ish: a substantial, interesting salad with heaps of leaves and some lean protein – perhaps smoked salmon or tuna or hummus. Throughout the day, I drink mineral water with a squeeze of lime, tons of herbal tea and plenty of black coffee. They just help the day tick by.

In my first four months on the Fast Diet, I lost 6kg, and my BMI went from 21.4 to 19.4. If you're struggling with bigger numbers than these, take strength from the fact that heavier subjects respond brilliantly to intermittent fasting, and the positive effects should be apparent in a relatively short time. These days, one fast a week (on Mondays) seems to suffice and keep me at a stable, happy weight.

Many women I encounter are well versed in dieting techniques (years of practice), and I've found that a couple of tips can come in handy on a Fast Day. I'd recommend, for instance, eating in small mouthfuls, chewing slowly and concentrating when eating. If you're only getting 500 calories, it makes sense to notice them as they go in.

I have found, like many intermittent fasters, that hunger is simply not an issue. For whatever reason – and one wonders whether it suits the food industry – we have developed a fear of hunger, fretting about low blood sugar and whatnot.

On the whole, for me, a day with little food feels

emancipating rather than restrictive. That said, there are ups and downs: some days skim by like a stone on water; other days, I feel like I'm sinking, not swimming, perhaps because emotions or hormones or simply the tricky business of life have kicked in. See how you feel, and always give in gracefully if that particular day is not your day to fast.

A dozen ways to make the Fast Diet work for you

1. *Know your weight, your BMI and your waist size from the get-go.* As we mentioned earlier, waist measurement is a simple and important gauge of internal fat and a powerful predictor of future health. BMI is your weight (in kilograms) divided by your height (in metres) squared; it may sound like a palaver, and an abstract one at that, but it's a widely accepted tool for plotting a path to healthy weight loss. Do note that a BMI score takes no account of body type, age or ethnicity, so should be greeted with informed caution. Still, if you need a number, this is a useful one.

Weigh yourself regularly but not obsessively. After the initial stages, once or twice a week should suffice. The mornings after Fast Days are best if you like to see falling figures. You may discover that your weight measurement is significantly different from day to day. This discrepancy may well be due to the additional weight of food in your system, rather than changes in your fat mass from one day to the next. You may like to take an average over several days to arrive at a reasonable figure for any weight loss. But don't overdo it; try not to make weighing – yourself or your calories – a chore.

2. *Chart your progress.* If you are someone who enjoys structure and clarity, you may want to monitor your progress (you'll find a helpful progress tracker on our website). Have a target in mind. Where do you want to be, and when? Be realistic: precipitous weight loss is not advised, so allow yourself time. Make a plan. Write it down. Aim to be specific: if you want to lose weight, there is a psychological advantage in setting a defined goal for how much weight you want to lose (10lb?) by when (15 March for your sister's wedding?)

Plenty of people recommend keeping a diet diary. Dieters who write daily notes are known to be more successful at losing weight than those who don't, with one study[37] finding that it can double weight loss as part of a managed programme. Logging consumption seems to heighten awareness; the simple act of quantifying incoming food (and, don't forget, drink) seems to strengthen your hand. Alongside the numbers and food notes, consider adding your Fast Day experiences; try to note three good things that happen each day. It's a feel-good message that you can refer to as time goes by. It helps too, in psychologists' jargon, to 'reframe the motivator'. Rather than thinking 'Arrgh, I don't want to be fat', focus on 'I'd like to be slimmer, healthier and full of energy'. Consider what you want, frame it positively, write it down, and read it every day.

3. *Find a fast friend.* You need very few accoutrements to make this a success, but a supportive friend may well be one of them. Once you're on the Fast Diet, tell people about it; you may find that they join in, and you'll develop a network of common experience. Since the plan appeals to men and women equally, couples report that they find it more manageable to do it together. That way, you get mutual support, camaraderie, joint commitment and shared anecdotes; besides, meal times are made infinitely easier if you're eating with someone who understands the rudiments of the plot. There are plenty of threads on online chat rooms too. Over the past two years, the 5:2 conversation has been evolving and growing online. To tune into the discussion, and to discover countless tips to make the Fast Diet work for you, go to thefastdiet. co.uk. Or investigate the many Facebook groups – ours is at www.facebook.com/thefastdiet.co.uk. It's remarkable how reassuring it is to know that you're not alone.

4. *Prep your Fast Day food in advance* so that you don't go foraging and come across a leftover sausage lurking irresistibly in the fridge. Shop and cook on non-Fast Days, so as not to taunt yourself with unnecessary temptation. Keep it simple, aiming for flavour without effort

(for simple, sustaining recipe ideas, see pages 169-212). Before you embark, undertake a spot of 'kitchen hygiene': clear the house of junk food. It will only croon and coo at you from the cupboards, making your Fast Day harder than it needs to be. Eliminate illicit food stashes; empty your snack drawer at work. And don't forget to check calorie labels for portion size. When the cereal box says 'a 30g serving', measure it. Go on. Be amazed. Then be honest. Since your calorie count on a Fast Day is necessarily fixed and limited, it's important not to be blinkered about how much is actually going in. You'll find a quick Calorie Counter on pages 230-33.

5. *Wait before you eat.* Try to resist for at least ten minutes, 15 if you can, to see if the hunger subsides (as it naturally tends to do). The idea here is to put food in its place. It's only food. Once you start to think about food in a rational and realistic way, you'll discover that you can modify your behaviour around it. You can even push it aside. You may discover, as many fasters attest, that you develop a keen sensitivity to your own appetite, hunger, satiety, digestion, metabolism. They will change from day to day. Stay quiet, and you can begin to feel these subtle, visceral things.

On Fast Days, eat with awareness, allowing yourself to fully absorb the fact that you're eating (not as daft as it sounds, particularly if you have ever sat in a traffic jam popping M&Ms). Similarly, on off-duty days, stay gently alert. Eat until you're satisfied, not until you're full (this will come naturally after a few weeks' practice). Work out what the concept of 'fullness' means for you – we are all different and it changes over time.

6. *Stay busy.* 'We humans are always looking for things to do between meals,' said Leonard Cohen. Yes, and look where it's got us. So fill your day, not your face. As fasting advocate Brad Pilon has noted, 'No one's hungry in the first few seconds of a sky dive.' Engage in things other than food – not necessarily sky diving, but anything that appeals to you. Distraction is your best defence against the dark arts of the food industry, which has stationed donuts on every street corner and nachos at every turn. And remember, if you absolutely must have that donut, it will still be there tomorrow.

7. *Experiment.* The key, as we've established, is to find a plan that works for you, which means you may need to experiment a little until you find your best fit for a sustainable, lifelong plan, not merely a short-lived practice. Rather than think of 5:2 as 'a diet', which in its modern usage is larded with quick-fix connotations, perhaps begin to see it as stemming from the classical Greek 'diaita'. This roughly translates as 'a manner of living'. A way of life. So, be playful. Customise.

8. *Don't be afraid to think about food you like.* A psychological mechanism called 'habituation' – in which the more people have of something, the less value they attach to it – means that doing the opposite and trying to suppress thoughts of food is probably a 'flawed strategy'.[38] The critical thought process here is to treat food as a friend, not as a foe. Food is not magical, supernatural or dangerous. Don't demonise it; normalise it. It's only food. Try not to associate fasting with discomfort; be gentle to cultivate the changes you desire; don't dwell on the downside if, say, a Fast Day is broken. Move on.

9. *Stay hydrated.* Find no-calorie drinks you like, and then drink them in quantity. Some swear by herbal tea; others prefer a mineral water with bubbles to dance on the tongue, though tap water will do just as well. Plenty of our hydration comes through the food we eat, so you may need to compensate with additional drinks beyond your routine intake (check your urine; it should be plentiful and pale). While there's no scientific rationale for drinking the recommended eight glasses of water a day, there is good reason to keep the liquids coming in. A dry mouth is the last sign of dehydration, not the first, so act before your body complains, recognising too that a glass of water is a quick way to hush an empty belly, at least temporarily. It will also stop you mistaking thirst for hunger.

10. *Don't count on weight loss on any given day.* If you have a week when the scales don't seem to shift, dwell instead upon the health benefits you will certainly be accruing even if you haven't seen your numbers drop. Remember why you're doing this: not just the smaller jeans, but the long-term advantages, the widely accepted disease-busting, brain-boosting, life-lengthening benefits of intermittent fasting. Think of it as a pension plan for your body. So keep your perspective: don't be disheartened if you 'plateau' in any given week; weight loss is your bonus, not your sole objective.

11. *Be sensible, exercise caution, and if it feels wrong, stop.* It's vital that this strategy should be practised in a way that's flexible and forgiving. If you're concerned about any aspect of intermittent fasting, see your doctor. Remember too that it's OK to break the rules if you need to. It's not a race to the finish, so be kind to yourself and make it fun.

12. *Congratulate yourself.* Every completed Fast Day means potential weight loss and quantifiable health gain. You're already winning. So? Say so. A study from the University of Chicago[39] reveals how positive feedback on new habits will increase the likelihood of success. Don't be afraid to grandstand your achievements. Website forums make an ideal platform for a bit of back-patting – go to thefastdiet.co.uk to see tons of support and praise in

action. Plenty of people on our site say that this is often enough to get them through a tricky patch.

Q & A

'Fasting is a fiery weapon. It has its own science. No one, as far as I'm aware, has a perfect knowledge of it.'

Gandhi

Which days should I choose to fast?

It really doesn't matter. It's your life, and you'll know which days will suit you best. Monday is an obvious choice for many, perhaps because it is more manageable, psychologically and practically, to gear yourself up at the beginning of a new week, particularly if it follows a sociable weekend. For that reason, fasters might choose to avoid Saturdays and Sundays, when family lunches and brunches, dinner dates and parties make calorie-cutting a chore. Thursday would then make a sensible second fasting day, chiming, if such things appeal, with the teachings of the Prophet Mohammed, who is understood to have fasted on the second and fifth days of the week. But be flexible; don't force yourself to fast when it feels wrong. If you're particularly stressed, off-colour, tired or peevish on a day that you have designated a fast, try again another day. Adapt. This is not about one-size-fits-all rules; it's about finding a realistic pattern that dovetails with your life. Do, however, aim for a pattern. That way, over time, your fasts will become familiar, a low-key habit you accept and embrace. You may adapt your fasts as your life (and your body) change shape – but don't drop too many Fast Days; there is a danger that you'll slide back into old habits. Be kind. But be tough.

When should I eat?

Go with a timetable that suits you. As we've seen, some fasters appreciate the convenience and simplicity of a single 500/600-calorie evening meal, allowing them to ignore food entirely for most of the day; some people say they actually feel hungrier during the day if they have breakfast. Having just one meal, as late in the day as possible, will clearly intensify the fast – allowing your body a longer period in which to enter a fasted state.

Others prefer to eat breakfast and then avoid food for a 'fasting window' of around 12 hours until supper. Since it is the fasted state that is so beneficial to us, eating lots of small meals is likely to reduce the benefits, particularly if you graze on carbohydrates. Remember that over time, as you get used to the diet, your body should acclimatise to periods of fasting; so keep your personal pattern flexible and adjust to a more lengthy fasting window when you feel able. Stay alert and tweak the regime to suit your needs.

WOMEN

FAST 500 MENU PLANS

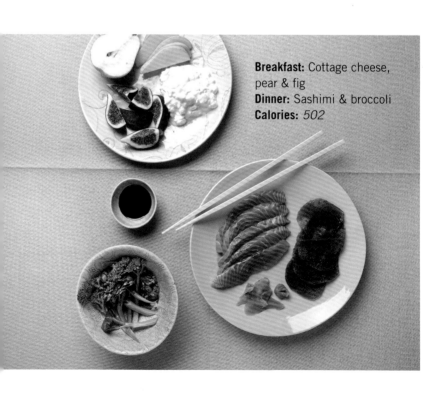

Breakfast: Cottage cheese, pear & fig
Dinner: Sashimi & broccoli
Calories: *502*

Breakfast: Porridge with blueberries **Dinner:** Chicken stir-fry, apple **Calories:** *505*

Breakfast: Poached egg, smoked salmon **Dinner:** Thai salad **Calories:** *496*

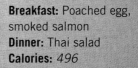

Breakfast: Strawberry smoothie
Dinner: Oven-baked smoked haddock
Calories: *490*

Breakfast: Dipped apple & mango
Dinner: Tuna bean salad
Calories: *502*

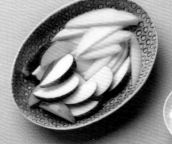

Breakfast: Ham, egg, tangerine
Dinner: Tortilla pizza, salad
Calories: *504*

Breakfast: Scrambled eggs, smoked salmon
Dinner: Warm vegetable salad, watermelon
Calories: *506*

MEN

FAST 600 MENU PLANS

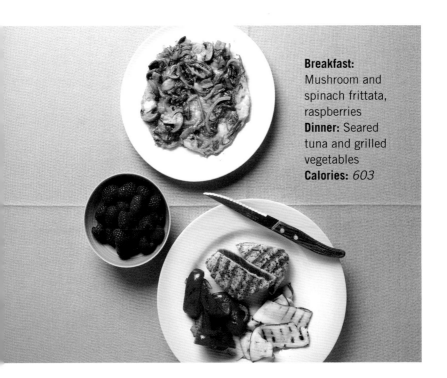

Breakfast: Mushroom and spinach frittata, raspberries
Dinner: Seared tuna and grilled vegetables
Calories: *603*

Breakfast: Poached eggs, grilled tomato
Dinner: Pesto salmon
Calories: *600*

Breakfast: Grilled kipper, 2 tangerines
Dinner: Steak with Asian coleslaw
Calories: *607*

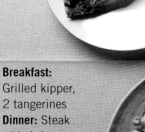

Breakfast: English breakfast
Dinner: Roast mackerel & veg
Calories: *603*

Breakfast: Yoghurt, nuts & fruit
Dinner: Turkey burger with corn on the cob
Calories: *612*

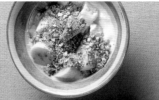

Breakfast: Yoghurt & muesli
Dinner: Roast pork with broccoli and cauliflower
Calories: *588*

Breakfast: Smoked salmon
Dinner: Bacon & butterbean soup, strawberries
Calories: *598*

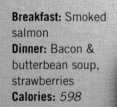

Does it have to be for 24 hours?

Fasting for a 'day' is practical, coherent and unambiguous, all of which will promise a greater chance of success. It is, however, merely the most convenient way of organising a fast: there's nothing magical about it. To save on bother, stick to the idea of a 'Fast Day', and remind yourself that you'll be asleep for nearly a third of it.

In reality, of course, a 'Fast Day', with its 500/600-calorie allowance, lasts up to 36 hours: if you finish your last full evening meal at 7.30pm on Sunday, and Monday is your Fast Day, you will eat normally again on Tuesday morning at around 7.30am. That is 36 hours. But don't get too particular about the numbers; the crux is that during a calendar 'day' your usual calorie consumption is slashed to a quarter.

Should I fast on consecutive days?

Some people like to fast on consecutive days, others prefer to have at least one day off between Fast Days. There are pros and cons.

If you do back-to-back fasts, your body will spend longer in the fasted state, which is generally speaking a good thing. Many people also like the pattern of, say, fasting on a Monday and Tuesday, ensuring that they get their two days over and done with, allowing them to relax for the rest of the week.

The danger, however, of fasting for two days in a row

is that you may start to feel resentful, bored and belea-guered – precisely the feelings that wreck the best-made diet intentions.

Michael tried the consecutive system and found it too challenging to be sustainable over time, so he switched to the split version – fasting on Mondays and Thursdays. The weight loss and the improvements in glucose, choles-terol and IGF-1 that he saw are all based on this non-consecutive, two-day pattern.

How much weight will I lose?

This will depend on your metabolism, your individual body type, your starting weight, your level of activity, how effectively and honestly you fast and how much you eat and drink on your non-Fast Days. Be judicious: abrupt weight loss is not advised and shouldn't be your aim: with rapid weight loss you will be losing a lot of muscle, which is not your goal.

In the Dublin study Michael mentioned earlier, which involved a combination of 5:2 and three short bursts of HIT (high intensity training) a week, there was an average weight loss of 4.6kg over 12 weeks, all of it fat.

In Dr Krista Varady's studies, where the subjects did the more intense ADF, they lost an average of between 3 and 5kg, almost all fat. Those who also did 40 minutes of exercise three times a week lost an average of 6.5kg.

In most intermittent fasting studies there is impressive fat loss around the gut, with 2-3 inches being lost around the waist.

What can I do if I'm not losing weight?

- Be patient. Some people will take longer than others to start losing weight. Remember to measure yourself around the waist, as what you really want to lose is fat

- Be realistic. Although some people lose a lot of weight straight off, the average is more like 1-2lb a week. It will happen

- Watch what you are eating on your non-Fast Days. The Fast Diet is not a free ticket to the all-u-can-eat buffet on the days when you're not fasting. Stay aware. Be sensible. Avoid bingeing. Yes, have treats, but make them a treat in the old-fashioned sense. These days, 'treats' are almost a food group in their own right; return them to their rightful place as occasional pleasures

- Keep a diary of everything you eat or drink for a week. Then look at the calorie content. Some foods may leap out. I was horrified to discover a muffin can be anywhere between 300 and 600 calories. And just because it says 'low fat' on the packet, it doesn't mean that it is low calorie. Some 'low-fat' foods (like muffins…) can contain more calories than the normal variety

- Look at the calories you are getting from drinks. Juices, lattes, alcohol, fizzy drinks, smoothies – they all contain a glut of calories. If you can graduate to drinking more water and sugar-free tea/coffee, it will help. Bear in mind that calories in drinks do not satiate: eat three apples and they will fill you up; drinking three apples in the form of a juice won't

- Moving more will certainly help. Michael always takes the stairs, even up seven flights. Get a pedometer and try to build up to doing 10,000 steps a day (most people do fewer than 5000). Exercise plus fasting will really help you keep the weight off. For more on incorporating exercise, see pages 82-89

- Try adding another Fast Day; go for a 4:3 pattern (four days normal eating, three days of reduced calories). Or you might consider ADF, particularly ADF plus exercise. In the study quoted above people doing ADF plus exercise lost, on average, 6.5kg (14lb) in 12 weeks

Will I go into starvation mode?

The short answer is an emphatic 'no'. This is one of the great dieting myths – the fear that if you cut your calories for even a day your metabolic rate will slow right down as your body tries to conserve its fat stores. This starvation mode myth seems to be based on the Minnesota starvation experiment, a study carried out during World War Two. In this experiment, young volunteers lived on extremely low-calorie diets for up to six months. The purpose of the study was to help scientists understand how to treat victims of mass starvation in Europe.

After prolonged starvation, when their body fat had fallen to less than 10%, there was a drop in body temperature and heart rate, suggesting that their basal metabolic rate (the energy burned by the body when at rest) had fallen. This, however, was an extreme situation.

A more recent experiment on the effects of short-term calorie restriction produced very different results. In this study, from the University of Vienna,[40] they took 11 healthy volunteers and asked them to live on nothing but water for 84 hours (in other words, a four-day fast). The researchers then measured the volunteers' metabolic rate at the end of each day. They found that their metabolic rates actually went up; after four days without food, they were 12% higher than at the beginning.

One reason for this may have been that they measured a significant rise in blood levels of a catecholamine called noradrenaline, which is known to burn fat. If they had continued the experiment, the volunteers' metabolic rates would eventually have fallen, not least because they would have begun to lose significant amounts of weight.

But, certainly in the short term, there is no evidence that starvation mode exists.

Indeed, when you think of it from an evolutionary perspective, 'starvation mode' makes little sense. Our remote ancestors often had to go without food for longish periods, and if, every time this happened, they had become less active and waited for pizza to be delivered they would have become extinct. Only during periods of prolonged famine would it make sense to slow the metabolism down and wait for better times to come.

Will my blood sugar fall, leaving me feeling faint?

In the trial mentioned above they also measured the volunteers' blood glucose levels. The researchers found that blood glucose levels did slowly fall over the three days, from 4.9mmol/l on day one to 3.5mmol/l by day four. These, however, are the sort of levels you might expect to see in a healthy person who had their blood taken before breakfast. They are not, in any sense, abnormally low. At the same time, the levels of fatty acids in their blood shot up, showing that their bodies had switched into major fat-burning mode.

Your body evolved to cope for periods without food. Intermittent fasting can be tough, but there is no evidence it will cause you to faint. If in reasonable good health, your body is a remarkably efficient and functional machine, capable of – in fact, designed for – the effective regulation of blood sugar. If you are diabetic, consult your doctor before embarking on any dietary change.

Will intermittent fasting lead to muscle breakdown?

Another fear is that intermittent fasting could lead to protein deficiency and muscle breakdown. It is true that the body doesn't store protein, so after 24 hours without any protein in your diet your body will seek amino acids for essential things like building your immune system by cannibalising existing muscle. But if your protein intake is adequate – and we actually recommend an increased protein percentage intake on Fast Days – then you are not going to get 'muscle protein breakdown'. In fact, the evidence from human studies suggests intermittent fasting is better than standard diets when it comes to muscle preservation.

I know I should stick to low GI foods on a Fast Day. So which foods are best?

As we've seen, foods with a low GI or GL will help keep your blood sugar stable, increasing your chances of a successful day with few calories. Vegetables and legumes are, needless to say, amazing, and you should rely on them on a Fast Day. Packed with nutrients, their bulk fills you up, they have relatively few calories and they keep your blood sugar low. Carrots are a great snack, particularly with hummus dip, which scores an astonishing GI of 6 and a GL of 0. Fruit is handy too, though some fruits are more fast-friendly than others. Check the GI count of your chosen Fast Day foods online. Diabetes UK has an excellent guide at www.diabetes.org.uk. Or look at the GI Index from the University of Sydney on www.glycemicindex.com, noting that some foods have an unexpected count. Staples, for instance, are worth scrutinising with an eagle eye:

STAPLES	GI	GL
BROWN RICE	48	20
WHITE RICE	76	36
PASTA durum wheat	40	20
COUSCOUS	65	23
POTATOES BOILED	58	16
MASHED	85	17
FRIED	75	22
BAKED	85	26

The biggest surprise regarding the staples is how great an effect baking or mashing potatoes has on blood sugars. On Fast Days, avoid these starchy basics, and substitute with plenty of greens. Fill your plate. Watch out for fruit too. Some are your fast friends; others will spike your blood sugar and are best left for the days when you are off duty.

FRUIT	GI	GL
STRAWBERRIES	38	1
APPLES	35	5
ORANGES	42	5

GRAPES	45	9
PINEAPPLE	84	7
BANANAS	50	12
RAISINS	64	30
DATES	100	42

Eating the whole fruit will keep you feeling full for longer. Strawberries, without sugar, are low GI/GL and also low calorie (no wonder many fasters eat a bowlful for breakfast). The striking thing to note is the high sugar impact of raisins and dates. Avoid them on Fast Days.

Beyond low-GI and protein foods, what else is on the 5:2 menu?

The following foods are tasty and low in calories, making them ideal for a Fast Day.

- VEGETABLES: When it comes to veg, the sky's the limit: it's hard to overdo your greens. But do apply the 5:2 mantra of the Double Vs – plenty of Volume, plenty of Variety. Aim to include different colours, textures, tastes, shapes. Steamed broccoli contains a whole world of nutrients (including vitamin K). Green beans love a little lemon and garlic. Fennel is great if shaved (invest in a mandolin), perhaps with orange segments and a squeeze of the juice. Edamame are a good source of low-fat protein and omega-3 fatty acids. Starchy veg, of course, tend to have a higher GL

and calorific value, though they are satiating. Proceed
with caution and don't add butter

- LEAVES: It goes without saying that green leafy veg
are your Fast Day friends. Spinach, kale, chard, salad
leaves… a veritable vit fest, and agreeably low
in calories. Pep things up with chilli flakes, ginger,
cumin, pepper, lemon juice, garlic

- FRUIT: Citrus fruits in general, and tangerines
in particular, contain high concentrations of
nobiletin, a compound that 'protects from obesity
and atherosclerosis' – in lab mice at least.[41] If you
like tangerines, eat them, perhaps spending time
meditatively peeling away the pith. The same group of
researchers previously found that grapefruit, rich in a
compound called naringenin, encourages the liver to
burn fat rather than store it.[42] Grapefruit also contains
compounds such as liminoids and lycopene (thought
to have anti-cancer properties),[43] and clocks in at
only 39 calories per half, making it a good Fast Day
food. (You should, however, be aware that grapefruit
interacts with a number of common medicines, so if
you are taking medication such as statins, consult
your doctor.) Alternatively, you could always throw in
a watermelon slice (30 calories per 100g) or an apple
(around 50 calories per 100g) for flavour, crunch and
pectin, a soluble fibre that can't be absorbed by the
body but is useful in fat digestion.[44] Apples are the

ultimate convenience food, though they are quite high in calories; eat the whole thing, skin, pips and core. Tomatoes also contain lycopene, which may help guard against cancer[45] and strokes.[46] A handful of cherry tomatoes or strawberries (low GI, low GL) could be your best bet to get you through a tummy rumble unscathed

- BERRIES: Blueberries are high in antioxidant polyphenols and phytonutrients. New research has found that they may also be able to break down fat cells in the body and prevent new ones from forming.[47] Even if you don't buy the science, blueberries remain a handy source of vitamin C

- NUTS: We've established that nuts are a Fast Day favourite: filling and low GI. Almonds, though calorific, are high in protein and fibre, which makes them brilliantly satiating; pistachios too (better yet, they take ages to crack and eat). Cashews and coconut flakes will help animate a salad. But count wisely: nut calories soon clock up

- CEREALS: Oats are a standby low-GL staple, but mix it up; you could experiment with bulgar, couscous or quinoa – the latter is high in protein and fibre, easy to cook and a good source of iron

- DAIRY: Milk products, though full of protein and calcium, can also be high in fat. Perhaps opt for low-fat alternatives – and save the cheeseboard for tomorrow. Fat-free or low-fat yoghurt contains protein, potassium (and, if you want them, pro-biotics), and, like nuts, it will help you feel fuller longer. But beware; flavoured varieties can also be high in sugar

- HERBS AND SPICES: Low-cal, high-impact, no brainer. Pickles may work for you too – cornichons, jalapeños, onions (watch the GI values) – or mustard; anything, really, that brings a bolt of fire or flavour to your plate

- SOUP: Scientists at Penn State University have found that soup is a great appetite suppressant.[48] Go for a light broth, rather than a meaty, creamy soup, to keep the calories in check

Whatever you eat on a Fast Day (or any day), the most important thing is to relish it. Go slow. Have a look at the menu plans on pages 169-91 and the recipes on pages 192-212 for more ideas; on pages 230-33, you'll find a quick Calorie Counter for 120 key Fast Day foods.

I know I need plenty of veg, but should I eat it raw or cooked?

There is some debate as to whether vegetables are best eaten raw or cooked; cooking may, as raw-foodists contend, destroy vitamins, minerals and enzymes, but it also softens cellulose fibres, making nutrients more available for take-up in the body. Lycopene, a potent antioxidant found in tomatoes, is boosted in cooking.[49] A small blob of ketchup is no bad thing. Meanwhile, boiled or steamed carrots, spinach, mushrooms, asparagus, cabbage, peppers and many other vegetables also supply more antioxidants, such as carotenoids and ferulic acid, to the body than they do when raw.[50] The downside of cooking veg is that it can destroy their vitamin C. The raw versus cooked argument is a complicated one. Our best advice? Eat plenty of vegetables, just the way you like them.

Can I eat what I like on off-duty days?

Counter-intuitive as it may seem, no foods are off-limits, none proscribed. On the five days a week when we're not restricting calories, we both occasionally eat fish and chips, roast potatoes, biscuits, cake.

The whole point of the 5:2 approach is that for five days a week you shouldn't feel as if you are on a diet. Even so, don't try to gorge in a bid to make up for lost time, like a contestant in a blueberry pie contest. You could compensate for fasting by grossly overeating the next day, but it's very hard to do and you probably won't want to. We are creatures of habit, which makes it difficult for us to change our ways. But ingrained habits can also be helpful – after a fast people seem to find it relatively easy to step back into normal eating.

This absence of 'hyperphagia' (excessive appetite) after

a day of rationing calories may seem surprising, but it is borne out by anecdotal experience. Many fasters report not feeling particularly hungry the day after a fast; what's more, many people discover that their life-long love of high-sugar, high-fat foods seems to diminish as intermittent fasting becomes a way of life. As yet, we can only speculate as to why this may be the case, but some individuals certainly experience a galvanising effect from the weight loss they achieve: as they drop the pounds, their resolve grows stronger and eating more healthily, cutting back on pizzas, pies and potatoes, seems a natural lifestyle change.

Humans have, however, evolved to prefer calorie-rich foods – it once gave us an edge – and perhaps the greatest advantage of the Fast Diet is that it allows 'pleasure foods', on five days of the week. For most of the time, there is no deprivation, no guilt. The psychological impact of not being denied is huge; it frustrates what's known as the 'disinhibition effect' – a paradox in which designating certain foods 'off-limits' makes us likely to eat more of them.[51]

Remember, then, that this is not a cycle of bingeing and starving: it is calibrated and moderate. Studies and experience show that intermittent fasting will regulate the appetite, not make it more extreme. You could pig out on your non-Fast Days, working your way steadily through all the ice-cream flavours in the freezer. (Even if you did, you'd still get some of the metabolic benefits of fasting.)

But you won't do that. In all likelihood, you'll remain gently, intuitively attentive to your calorie intake, almost without noticing.

Similarly, you may find yourself naturally favouring healthier foods once your palate is modified by your twice-weekly fasts. So, yes, eat freely, forbid nothing, but trust your body to say 'when'. In short, on a non-Fast Day:

- Eat until 'reasonably full'

- If you want one, include the occasional treat

Is breakfast vital?

Dieting lore has long suggested that breakfast is the most important meal of the day – miss it in the morning and it's like leaving the house without a coat. But is it true?

One way to find out is to take two groups of people, breakfast skippers and breakfast eaters, and make them swap habits. In a recent study, researchers did just that.[52] They recruited 300 overweight volunteers and asked the breakfast skippers to eat breakfast, while those who routinely ate breakfast were asked to skip it. There was high compliance with the new regimes; so what actually happened?

Well, the habitual breakfast skippers who had made themselves eat breakfast lost an average of 0.76kg. That is not a huge amount, but it is consistent with what breakfast advocates might expect. Except that the habitual breakfast eaters, who had spent 16 weeks skipping breakfast, lost an almost identical amount – an average of 0.71kg. The researchers concluded that, contrary to widely held belief, eating breakfast 'had no discernible effect on weight loss in free-living adults who were attempting to lose weight'.

If you are one of those people who doesn't like eating breakfast and who, perhaps, finds that eating breakfast first thing makes you hungrier, there seems to be no compelling scientific reason to make yourself eat it.

What can I drink on a Fast Day?

Plenty – as long as it doesn't have a substantial calorie content. In practice, as with most decisions on the Fast Diet, the choice is entirely up to you. Drink lots of water – it's calorie-free, actually free, more filling than you think and will stop you confusing thirst for hunger. In summer, add rounds of cucumber or a dash of lime. Freeze it and suck on ice cubes. If you want warmth, miso soup contains protein, feels like food and clocks up only 84 calories per cup; vegetable bouillon pulls off the same trick. If you find it hard to sleep, a mug of instant low-cal hot chocolate is under 40 calories and a comforting thought.

During the day no-cal drinks are best. Hot water with lemon is a standby favourite for fasters, but you might prefer to add mint leaves or a scattering of cloves, a slice of ginger root or some lemongrass. If you are fond of herbal teas, try some unfamiliar flavours to spice up the day (liquorice and cinnamon, lemon grass and ginger, lavender, rose and chamomile...) Try fruit teas chilled from the fridge. Green tea may have health-giving anti-oxidant properties (the jury's out), but if you like it, drink it.

On Fast Days we drink our tea and coffee black and sugarless; if you prefer it with milk and artificial sweeteners, fine. A small glass of milk is in fact a healthier drink than, say, orange juice, being rich in protein and relatively low in carbohydrates. But beware that the calories in milk add up, and what you are trying to do is extend the time you are not consuming any calories at all.

While fruit juices are seen as healthy, they generally have a surprisingly high sugar content, are lower in fibre than a whole fruit and can rack up the stealth calories without so much as a by-your-leave. Commercial smoothies can have a similar sugar content to Coke and, because they are acidic, they are corrosive to your teeth; they are also loaded with calories. If you need flavour, swap juice and smoothies for very dilute cordials – perhaps a dash of elderflower with fizzy water and lots of ice.

Can I have Diet Coke?

If it's the only thing that sustains you and your temper during a fast, then fine. But, counter-intuitive as it may seem, studies suggest that consuming zero-calorie sweeteners such as those found in diet drinks *increases* the risk of putting on weight[53] because they provide an 'orosensory stimulus' which convinces the body that a deluge of calories is about to come its way. When the advertised calories don't materialise, the system becomes confused – and as a result 'people eat more or expend less energy than they otherwise would'. The findings are open to debate: perhaps the best approach would be to limit intake, opting sometimes for sparkling water instead.

What about alcohol?

Alcoholic drinks, though pleasant, merely provide 'empty' calories. One glass of white wine contains about 120, while a 550ml can of beer has 250. Unless you really can't say no, abstain absolutely on a Fast Day – it's a golden opportunity to slash your weekly consumption without feeling serially deprived. Think of it as an alcovoid, for two achievable days each week.

And caffeine?

There's a growing body of evidence to suggest that – far from being a guilty pleasure – drinking coffee may be good for you, helping to prevent mental decline, improve cardiac health and reduce the risk of liver cancer and strokes.[54] So go ahead, drink coffee if that's what gets you going and keeps you going each day. It's a useful weapon in your arsenal against boredom, and coffee breaks can pleasantly punctuate your day. There's no metabolic reason to avoid caffeine during a fast, but if you have trouble sleeping, limit your intake later in the day. You should, of course, drink it black. A 16 fl oz caramel macchiato has 224 calories…

How about snacks?

The general idea of the Fast Diet is to give your body an occasional holiday from eating. Let your mouth rest. Give your belly a break. All calories count on a Fast Day, and your objective is to achieve as long a fasting window as possible. Having a complete moratorium on snacking, though challenging, actually makes the process easier to handle: if 'no means no', then you avoid questions or calorie calculations. No nibbles, no quibbles.

If you absolutely must snack on a Fast Day, do it with awareness and frugality: choose something that will not serve to elevate your insulin levels. Try a few apple slices or some strawberries. Try carrot or celery sticks with hummus, or a handful of nuts – always factoring them into your daily calorie count (don't cheat); for a full list of fast-friendly snacks, see page 211. And always keep an eye on the GI:

	GI	GL
NUTS	27	3
POPCORN	72	8

RICE CAKES	80	19
FRUIT BARS	93	20
MARS BAR	65	26

You knew that chocolate bars were hardly a health food, but did you know how sugary rice cakes and fruit bars can be? Bear in mind that processed foods tend to have hidden sugars and, though convenient, won't give you anything like the nutritional advantage of good old-fashioned plants and proteins.

Habitual snacking, even on low-calorie, nutrient-rich foods, is not advised; part of the motive here is to retrain your appetite, so don't overstimulate it. If your mouth is desperate for attention, give it a drink.

Can I use meal-replacement shakes to get me through the early days?

A number of people say that commercially available meal-replacement shakes helped them through the first, and normally hardest, weeks of an intermittent fast. Arguably, shakes are simpler than calorie-counting, and on your Fast Day you could simply sip away when waves of hunger strike. We are not great fans as we think real food is better. But if you find it helps, by all means try it. It's best to go for brands that are low in sugar.

What are the implications of cheating and having a few crisps or a cookie?

To clarify: this is a book about fasting, the voluntary abstention from eating food. The reasons why this is good for you go way beyond the fact that you are simply eating fewer calories. They arise because our bodies are designed for intermittent fasts. As you've seen, what does not kill you makes you stronger. So while starvation is bad, a little bit of short, sharp, shock food restriction is good.

Your aim, then, is to carve out a food-free breathing space for your body. Going to 510 calories (or 615 for a man) won't hurt – it won't obliterate a fast. Indeed, the idea of slashing calories to a quarter of your daily intake on a Fast Day is simply one that has been proven to have systemic effects on the metabolism. While there's no particular 'magic' to 500 or 600 calories, do try to stick to these numbers; you need clear parameters to make the strategy effective in the medium term.

Having a cookie on a Fast Day would be antithetical to your goals (not to mention the fact that it would probably spike your blood sugar and eat up most of your allowance in one buttery bite); when you're fasting, you need to think sensibly and coherently about your food choices, following the plan laid out here. Exercise willpower, reminding yourself that tomorrow is on its way.

What tests can I do to monitor changes?

Weigh yourself, of course, and measure your waist, chest and hips once or twice a week, keeping a note of progress (you'll find a simple tracker on our website). Some weighing machines will also give you an estimate of your body fat. You could also take a measure of your resting pulse, particularly if you are combining 5:2 with exercise, as this is a good predictor of future health. You could ask your doctor to measure fasting glucose and cholesterol, and take your blood pressure.

Will I get enough nutrients in my diet?

Yes. Remember: you fast only for short periods, only twice a week. During this time, you'll eat satiating and nutritious foods, low in fat and sugar. If you stick to the tenets of the Fast Diet, eating reasonably and normally on non-Fast Days, your diet should be nutritionally sound.

Should I take supplements during my fast?

The Fast Diet is an intermittent method, not a deprivation regime, so your nutritional intake from a wide variety of food sources should remain relatively steady over time, providing all the vitamins and minerals you require. If, as recommended, your Fast Day foods centre on protein and plants, they'll give you all the goodness you need so you won't have to resort to costly bottled multivitamins. Do, however, choose your Fast Day foods with care, ensuring that, over the course of a week, you consume adequate B vitamins, omega 3s, calcium and iron. Be sensible and eat well. While we are not fans of bottled vitamins and minerals, if a qualified health professional has suggested a particular supplement, you should continue to take it.

I've read about 'super-foods' and 'intelligent eating'. Should I include super-foods during a Fast Day?

The term 'super-food' is more of a marketing ploy than a scientific construct, and clinical nutritionists are loath to use the description. All plants produce a huge range of phytochemicals that can have a beneficial role in the body: eat them on a Fast Day or, indeed, on any day you please.

Should I exercise on a Fast Day?

Why not? As you will have gathered by now, we Fast Dieters are also keen on Fast Exercise. Research has shown that even a more extreme three-day total fast has no negative effect on the ability to perform short-term, high intensity workouts or long-duration, moderate intensity exercise. Athletes seem to suffer no loss in performance during occasional fasting; a 2008 study of Tunisian footballers during Ramadan found that fasting had no effect on performance ('Each player was assessed for speed, power, agility, endurance, and for passing and dribbling skills. No variables were negatively affected by fasting.')[55]

In fact – and this is worth noting if you are aiming for optimal fitness – training while fasting can result in better metabolic adaptations[56] (which means enhanced performance over time), improved muscle protein synthesis,[57] and a higher anabolic response to post-exercise feeding.[58]

Training on an empty stomach turns out to be beneficial on multiple levels, coaxing the body to burn a greater percentage of fat for fuel instead of relying on recently consumed carbs; if you're burning fat, don't forget, you're not storing it. As we've seen, one recent study found that working out before breakfast is beneficial for metabolic performance and weight loss.[59] A report in *The New York Times* suggested that it even 'blunts the deleterious effects of over-indulging' – making fasted exercise a canny way of 'combating Christmas'.[60] According to the study's authors, 'Our current data indicate that exercise training in the fasted state is more effective than exercise in the carbohydrate-fed state.' Certainly food for thought.

Do not, however, increase your Fast Day food allowance to 'compensate' for calories burned through exercise: on a Fast Day, stick to 500 or 600 calories, whatever level of activity you choose. That's where the benefits lie.

Are there gender differences in response to intermittent fasting?

Clearly, men and women have metabolic and hormonal differences; for evolutionary reasons, we store and utilise fat in different ways. Women carry more fat, are better at storing it and tend to be more efficient at burning it in response to exercise.[61] Though few studies have been done, there's some evidence to suggest that fasting women have a better response to endurance training than weight training,[62] while men may fare better with weights. Anecdotally, men tend to find working out on an empty stomach easier to accomplish than women.

In terms of general health, the benefits of intermittent fasting for both sexes are pretty clear. Although quite a few studies have been done with male volunteers, others have been done with a mixed group or mainly female volunteers. The volunteers who took part in Michelle Harvie's studies, well over 200 of them, were all women. Their results are striking and positive; nevertheless, further trials are required to analyse the precise effects of fasting on hormones, particularly among women of different ages. As with all recommendations in this book, be cautious and self-aware. This is not meant to be a struggle; it's intended as a well-marked route to good health. If, for whatever reason, short bouts of fasting interrupt your cycle or your sleep pattern, modify your approach till you find a comfortable balance that works for you.

Should I fast during my period?

Some women may find fasting more challenging on the days preceding a period; not enough research has been carried out on the impact of intermittent fasting on the menstrual cycle, but if you feel this may be the case for you, perhaps embark in the days following the start of your period, rather than before.

Can I fast if I'm trying to get pregnant?

The science is still unfolding, and there haven't been enough clinical trials to assess the overall effects of fasting on fertility. According to Professor Mark Mattson, an intermittent fasting plan, such as the Fast Diet, will not affect fertility. More extreme fasting may. It does in animals, but in a reversible manner. Nonetheless, we err on the side of caution and suggest that if you are trying to get pregnant, you should not fast.

Who else shouldn't fast?

There are certain groups for whom fasting is not advised. These are:

- Children: they are still growing and should not be subject to nutritional stress of any kind

- Type 1 diabetics and diabetics on insulin

- Pregnant women and breast-feeding mothers, who should eat according to government guidelines and not limit their calorie intake

- Anyone with an eating disorder, and the very lean or underweight

- People recovering from surgery, and those with an underlying medical condition or taking prescribed medications: we would advise you to see your doctor first, as you would before embarking on any weight-loss regime

- Anyone feeling unwell or feverish: fasting will stress your body which, as we've seen, is one of the reasons that it is effective (as stress provokes repair), but you shouldn't *over*stress

- People taking warfarin: consult your doctor first as it may increase your INR

Will I get headaches?

If you do, it may be due to dehydration rather than a lack of calories. You might experience mild withdrawal symptoms from sugar (or caffeine if you've dropped it), but the brevity of your fast shouldn't make this of particular concern. Keep drinking water. Treat a headache as you would normally; if fasting today is making you feel really unwell, stop. You are in charge.

Will I become constipated?

If constipation is an issue, it's often the result of not drinking enough water. So stay hydrated. Try adding psyllium husk to your diet. If the problem persists, consult your GP.

Will I feel tired?

Short-term, deliberate, modified fasting should not exhaust you – some fasters even report an energy boost on a Fast Day and beyond. As in normal life, you'll undoubtedly have up days and down days, good days and bad. See how you fare. You may find that a Fast Day ends earlier than usual – an absence of alcohol and plentiful sleep being a great way to arrive at breakfast sooner.

Will I feel cold?

Some people, my father included, do report feeling a bit cold after losing weight on the 5:2. If you have carried a fair amount of weight around for many years, almost as a comfort blanket, losing it will certainly have an effect. You could do some energetic exercise to stoke things up. Or wear an extra sweater…

Will I go to bed hungry?

Probably not, though it will depend on your particular

metabolism, and how you timed your Fast Day calorie consumption. If you feel hungry, take your mind off it – a bubble bath, a good book, a stretch out, a herbal tea. Get psychology on your side: congratulate yourself on reaching the end of another Fast Day. Surprisingly, perhaps, fasters report that they don't wake up ravenous and run to the fridge as soon as the alarm goes off. Hunger is a subtle beast, and your appetite will soon find its rhythm.

Will fasting affect my sleep?

Some people find it hard to sleep on a relatively empty stomach. If so, Michael recommends setting aside calories for a late-night glass of milk or small snack. There is evidence that the side effects you experience are the ones you expect, so it is best to approach intermittent fasting with the expectation that it will be fine.

Will fasting affect my gout?

Longer-term fasting can precipitate gout, but this should not occur with intermittent fasting. In fact, gout is associated with metabolic syndrome (obesity, insulin resistance, high cholesterol, high blood pressure) and 5:2 should help correct this, partly through weight loss but also by reducing insulin levels. In addition, as Michael has outlined above, intermittent fasting seems to reduce inflammation.

What if everyone around me is eating on one of my Fast Days?

Participate, but with a nonchalant awareness. While support from family and friends is an asset, making a song and dance about your fast will only cause you to feel self-conscious, turning the diet into an obstruction, a hurdle, rather than something that should slot happily and calmly into your life. Remember your trump card: you'll eat normally again tomorrow. Some days, of course, are tougher than others. Naturally enough, you may find yourself feeling hungrier and less able to fast successfully when celebrating or attending events which revolve around food.

If you know that you have a social event in the diary, fast the day before or the day after. The flexibility of the plan explicitly means – in fact, it demands – that you still go to that wedding, birthday, anniversary dinner, christening, bar mitzvah, supper date, posh restaurant. Take a break for Christmas, Easter, Thanksgiving, Diwali. Yes, you may well put on a little weight, but this is a life, not a life sentence. You can always deviate, eat chips and dips and things on sticks, and then revert to more challenging fasting once the party's over.

What if I'm currently obese?

Clinical trials have concluded that intermittent fasting is a sustainable – indeed, one of the most effective – ways for obese individuals to lose weight and keep it off; the larger you are, the greater your initial weight loss is likely to be. If you are obese it's likely that, for whatever reason, traditional restrictive diets have failed for you. The Fast Diet is different because of its flexibility, its war on guilt, and its approval of occasional 'pleasure foods' on non-Fast Days. Studies by Dr Michelle Harvie and Professor Tony Howell, cited above, have shown that most overweight women are able to adapt to calorie restricting two days a week and lose significant amounts of fat, even those who have had long-term weight issues. As with any underlying medical condition, we recommend that you fast under supervision.

Should I add a third day if I want to see accelerated results, and do 4:3?

As Michael wrote earlier, there is good scientific evidence from trials run by Dr Krista Varady and her team at the University of Illinois in Chicago of benefits from more rigorous intermittent fasting. They have done a number of carefully controlled studies where volunteers have tried ADF. This form of intermittent fasting entails cutting calories every other day – a 500-calorie allowance for women, 600 for men. Most volunteers who took part in these studies lost significant amounts of weight, mainly as fat, and saw marked improvements in their biomarkers, including cholesterol.

I'm already slim enough, but would like to enjoy the health benefits of intermittent fasting. Is that possible?

If you are already at a reasonable, happy weight, you can still fast effectively, but consider adapting your consumption on non-Fast Days to encompass more calorie-dense foods. The main researchers we talked to in this field are all slim and they still fast. With practice, you will discover an amicable balance between fasting and feeding which keeps your weight in the prescribed range. As you reach your target weight, alter your routine to fast once a week, rather than twice a week. This is what we call the Maintenance Model, or 6:1.

While there have been no specific studies to illuminate the effects of fasting for one day, it seems likely that it will provide similar benefits, beyond weight loss, as fasting for two. We know, for example, that repair and routine maintenance goes on in the cells when we are not eating; studies suggest that a day a week of calorie restriction will keep the weight off and allow you to retain significant biochemical benefits.

So, use your common sense and watch the scales; don't slide. As mentioned above, if you are already extremely lean or suffering from an eating disorder, fasting of any description is not advised. If in doubt, see your GP.

Is it too late to start?

On the contrary, there's no time to lose. The Fast Diet is

likely to prolong your life. It will moderate your appetite and help you lose weight. Its effects are quickly felt, often within a week of starting your simple bi-weekly mini fasts. It all points to a healthier, leaner, longer old age, fewer doctors' appointments, more energy, greater resistance to disease. Our advice? Start yesterday.

How long should I continue?

Interestingly, the Fast Diet's On/Off eating scheme looks a lot like the approach of many naturally slim people. Some days they'll pick, other days they'll tuck into treats. In the long run, this is how the Fast Diet goes. As you settle into the routine, you'll naturally moderate your calorie intake on Fast Days and feed days, until the process is innate. When you reach your target weight, you can change the frequency of your fast. Play with it. But don't drift; stay alert.

Your aim is a permanent life change, not a blip, not a fad, not a dinner-party chat. This is a long-distance route to sustained weight loss. Accept that it is something you will do, in a form that suits you, indefinitely. For as long as life.

The future of fasting: where next?

Fasting, as we mentioned at the beginning of the book, has been practised for many thousands of years and yet science is only just starting to catch up. The first evidence of the long-term benefits of calorie restriction were found just over 80 years ago, when nutritionists working with rats at Cornell University in the US discovered that if you severely restrict the amount they eat, they live longer. Much longer.

Since then, the evidence has continued to mount that animals not only live longer, healthier lives if they are calorie-restricted, they also do so if they are intermittently starved. In recent years the research has moved on from rodents to humans and we are seeing the same patterns of improvement.

So where do we go from here? Professor Valter Longo, who has done so much pioneering work with IGF-1, is running a number of human trials in conjunction with colleagues at the University of Southern California, looking at the impact of fasting on cancer. They have already demonstrated that fasting will cut your risk of developing cancer; now they want to see if fasting will also improve the efficacy of chemotherapy and radiotherapy.

Valter Longo believes that we should try to tackle the problems of ageing as a whole, rather than one disease at a time. Instead of focusing so much research money on heart disease or cancer, we should try to slow down the cellular damage that leads to the diseases of old age. Fasting, whether short term or intermittent, is clearly one way to do this.

Dr Michelle Harvie and Professor Tony Howell, who work at the Genesis Breast Cancer Prevention Centre in Manchester, have done a great deal of fascinating work developing and testing different forms of two-day intermittent energy restriction. In this book we have quoted a couple of their studies – involving hundreds of female volunteers – which have shown that people can lose weight just as effectively by calorie restricting on an intermittent basis as by calorie restricting every day. They are planning further studies, comparing what they call 'The 2-Day Diet' with standard dieting. These studies will undoubtedly add to our understanding of how well people are able to tolerate different patterns of eating in the long run.

Professor Mark Mattson of the National Institute on Aging in Baltimore is adding all the time to the dozens of research papers he has already published on the effects of fasting and intermittent fasting on the brain. We are particularly interested to see the outcome of some of his current studies, which include looking further into what happens to the brains of volunteers when put on an intermittent fasting regime.

He is keen to emphasise the importance of regular exercise alongside intermittent fasting, as many of the changes he sees, whether it's improving glucose regulation or the effects on the brain, are similar with exercise and intermittent fasting. Any form of exercise is better than nothing, but there is currently a lot of excitement around HIT (high intensity training), which seems to produce greater changes in less time.

Despite the benefits, many people may not want to fast, so there is considerable interest in developing drugs that mimic some of the effects of intermittent fasting. There is a drug called Byetta, used for the treatment of diabetes, which also activates the production of BDNF (brain-derived neurotrophic factor). This in turn, as we've seen, seems to protect the brain against the ravages of ageing. The hope is that Byetta or a related drug will, if not prevent dementia, at least significantly slow its progression.

Another interesting candidate is the drug rapamycin, first isolated from bacteria found in the soil of Easter Island. Rapamycin, like fasting, acts on something called the mTor pathway, which regulates protein synthesis and cell growth. It is implicated in a range of common diseases, including diabetes, obesity, depression and some cancers. Pharmaceutical companies are currently creating and testing modified versions of rapamycin.

Intermittent fasting has, until now, been one of the best-kept secrets in science. We look forward, with a great deal of personal interest, to seeing how this particular story unfolds.

THE FAST DIET EATING PLAN

Fast Day cooking tips

1. Feel free to bump up the quantities of leafy, low-calorie, low-GI vegetables. It is difficult to pig out on leafy veg, and if you need bulk, here's where you should get it. Lightly steaming veg is the best cooking method, so invest in a tiered bamboo steamer, and cook your proteins and veggies in several health-packed, eco-friendly levels. Scrub vegetables rather than peel them, as many nutrients are found close to the skin. Eating the skins will add fibre to your diet. When browning and caramelising vegetables, put them in a hot, dry pan and then spray with oil, rather than adding the oil first – this will reduce the amount of oil absorbed during cooking.

2. Some vegetables benefit from cooking, others are better eaten raw. See page 140 for more details. Cooking certain veg – including carrots, spinach, mushrooms, asparagus, cabbage and peppers – breaks down the cell structure without destroying vitamins, allowing you to

absorb more goodies. For raw vegetables, a mandolin makes preparation easy and swift.

3. Fast Days should be low fat, rather than no fat. A teaspoon of olive oil can be used in cooking or drizzled over vegetables for flavour; or use a cooking-oil spray to get a thin film. Alternatively, use a silicon brush to apply oil to the pan and dab away excess with kitchen paper. Do include a light oil dressing on your salads; it means that you are more likely to absorb their fat-soluble vitamins.

4. Always cook with a non-stick pan to cut down on calorie-dense fats. Add a splash of water if the food sticks.

5. The acid in lemon or orange dressings means that you will absorb more iron from leafy greens such as spinach and kale. Watercress with orange is a great combination, perhaps scattered with some sesame and sunflower seeds or blanched almonds, for a little protein and crunch.

6. Eating protein will help keep you fuller longer. Stick to the low-fat proteins, including some nuts and legumes. Cooking meat and poultry with its skin on will maximise flavour and prevent drying out, but don't eat the skin. Much of the fat lies there. Roast it on a rack over a baking pan to allow excess fat to drip away. Similarly, a griddle

pan channels fat into the grooves and away from your plate.

7. Swap minced beef for mushrooms or Quorn to lessen your calorie load, and consider extending your meat eating to include lean game. Venison, for example, has a fraction of the fat found in beef. Eggs, meanwhile, are a Fast Day stand-by; boiling or poaching them means you're not adding further calories.

8. Dairy is also included here: choose lower-fat cheeses and semi-skimmed milk, and avoid full-fat yoghurts in favour of low-fat alternatives. Drop the lattes and bin the butter on a Fast Day: they are calorie traps.

9. Avoid starchy white carbohydrates (bread, potatoes, pasta) and opt instead for low-GI carbs such as vegetables, pulses and slow-burn cereals. Choose brown rice and quinoa. Porridge for breakfast will keep you fuller for longer than a commercial cereal.

10. Ensure that you get some fibre in your fast: eat the skin of apples and pears, have oats for breakfast, keep those leafy vegetables coming in.

11. Add flavour where you can: chilli flakes will give a kick to any savoury dish. Vinegars, including balsamic, and

lemon juice will lend acidity. Add fresh herbs too – they are virtually calorie-free, but give personality to a plate.

12. Soup can be a saviour on a hungry day, particularly if you choose a light broth packed with leafy veg (a Vietnamese pho would be ideal, though hold back on the noodles). Soup is satiating, and a good way of using up ingredients languishing in the fridge. When making a soup base, don't sweat veg in butter; use water or a spray of oil. Thicken with pulses instead of potatoes (a handful of lentils will do the trick), or gravitate towards clear vegetable broths; veg stock generally has a lower fat content than chicken stock. If it suits the recipe, leave veggies whole rather than blitzing. Add miso, stock cubes or bouillon powder to capitalise on taste.

13. Use agave as a sweetener if required; it's relatively low-GI. Or try Stevia.

14. Unless otherwise specified, weigh your food after preparing it, so that the calorie count is correct.

FAST 500 MENU PLANS FOR WOMEN

DAY 1

Breakfast *174 calories*
½ tub of low-fat cottage cheese (100g, 100 calories)
½ small pear (100g, 50 calories)
1 fresh fig (50g, 24 calories)

Dinner *328 calories*
Sashimi: 3-5 pieces salmon (100g, 185 calories) and tuna
(90g, 120 calories) – served with soy sauce, wasabi and
ginger, and tenderstem broccoli topped with ½ tsp olive oil
(20 calories), squeeze of lemon and slices of fresh red chilli
(3 calories)

Daily total: 502 calories

DAY 2

Breakfast *175 calories*
Simple porridge made with 40g jumbo oats (155 calories) and 200ml water. Top with 30g blueberries (20 calories)

Dinner *330 calories*
Chicken stir-fry: cut chicken fillet into strips (120g, 175 calories). Spray a non-stick pan with olive oil (10 calories) and fry chicken with 1 tsp finely chopped ginger (2 calories), 1 tbsp chopped coriander (3 calories), a clove of crushed garlic (3 calories), 2 tsp soy sauce (3 calories) and ½ squeezed lemon (1 calorie) until browned and sealed, adding water if chicken sticks. Add a handful of sugar snap peas (15g, 12 calories), 100g finely sliced cabbage (26 calories) and 1 carrot cut into thin strips (120g, 45 calories), and cook for 5-10 more mins or until the chicken is cooked, adding water if necessary. Season and serve

1 apple (50 calories)

Daily total: 505 calories

DAY 3

Breakfast *130 calories*
1 large boiled egg (90 calories)
½ small grapefruit (115g, 40 calories)

Dinner *371 calories*
Vegetarian chilli: fry a chopped clove of garlic (3 calories)
and ½ finely chopped red chilli (1 calorie) in 1 tsp olive oil
(40 calories). Add a pinch of cumin and 1 large or 4 small
chopped mushrooms (20g, 3 calories) and cook for 5 mins,
adding water if it sticks. Add ½ tin of chopped tomatoes
(200g, 44 calories) and ½ tin of kidney beans (120g, 180
calories), stir, season and simmer for 10-15 mins. Serve with
2 tbsp cooked wild brown rice (80g, 100 calories)

Daily total: 501 calories

DAY 4

Breakfast *220 calories*
Smoked salmon (75g, 140 calories) and a poached egg (80 calories)

Dinner *276 calories*
Thai salad: put 1 tbsp Thai fish sauce (10 calories), the juice of ½ lime (20g, 2 calories), ½ tsp sugar (8 calories), 2 sliced spring onions (20g, 5 calories) and 1 red chilli, finely chopped (1 calorie) into a bowl. Mix well. Add 20 small cooked prawns (60g, 60 calories), 1 large carrot, julienned (150g, 70 calories) and 70g vermicelli noodles (100 calories), soaked according to instructions. Season, toss well and serve with handful of leaf salad (10 calories) dressed with a spray of olive oil and squeeze of lemon juice (10 calories)

Daily total: 496 calories

DAY 5

Breakfast *175 calories*
<u>Strawberry smoothie:</u> blend a small banana (90g, 83 calories), a pot of fat-free natural yoghurt (150g, 62 calories), a large handful of strawberries (100g, 30 calories), a splash of water and some ice until thick and creamy. Serve immediately

Dinner *315 calories*
<u>Oven-baked smoked haddock:</u> place a fillet of smoked haddock (200g, 202 calories) on a non-stick baking tray and roast for 15–20 mins, or until fish is cooked through. Serve with a large poached egg (90 calories) and lightly steamed baby leaf spinach (100g, 23 calories)·

Daily total: 490 calories

DAY 6

Breakfast *245 calories*
Dipped apple and mango: slice 1 small apple (100g, 50 calories) and 1 mango (160g, 95 calories) and serve with 2 tbsp half-fat crème fraîche 'dip' (100 calories)

Dinner *257 calories*
Tuna bean salad: put 140g tinned cannellini beans (110 calories), 120g good-quality canned tuna in spring water (114 calories), 8 chopped cherry tomatoes (90g, 16 calories), 2 tsp chopped red onion (6 calories) and a generous handful of baby leaf spinach (30g, 8 calories) in a salad bowl. Mix well. Drizzle over a dressing made from ½ clove of crushed garlic (2 calories), the juice and zest of 1 lemon (1 calorie), salt and pepper and a splash of white wine vinegar

Daily total: 502 calories

DAY 7

Breakfast *150 calories*
1 small boiled egg (75 calories)
1 slice of ham (40g, 50 calories)
1 tangerine (80g, 25 calories)

Dinner *354 calories*
Tortilla pizza: take 1 tortilla (55g, 144 calories) and top with 2 tbsp passata (5 calories), torn pieces of light mozzarella (80g, 130 calories), and scatter with chopped vegetables: mushrooms, red pepper, courgette, red onion and aubergine (170g, 50 calories). Season and cook in a hot oven for 5-10 mins. Serve topped with fresh basil leaves and a side salad of leaves drizzled with a spray of olive oil (25 calories).

Daily total: 504 calories

DAY 8

Breakfast *231 calories*
<u>Scrambled eggs:</u> add 1 tbsp skimmed milk (15g, 5 calories)
to 2 small beaten eggs (150 calories), season and scramble
in a non-stick frying pan (no added oil or butter). Chop 40g
smoked salmon (76 calories) and stir into the eggs

Dinner *275 calories*
<u>Warm vegetable salad:</u> mix 10 cherry tomatoes (120g, 22
calories),.with ½ a sliced courgette (75g, 16 calories), ½ a
sliced aubergine (120g, 25 calories), 1 sliced red pepper
(160g, 50 calories). Scatter with basil leaves (1 calorie) and
drizzle with 1 tsp balsamic vinegar (5 calories). Roast in
a hot oven for 20–25 mins. Season and serve with 2 tbsp
Parmesan (20g, 90 calories)

200g watermelon (66 calories)

Daily total: 506 calories

DAY 9

Breakfast *147 calories*
1 small pot of fat-free natural yoghurt (150g, 62 calories)
50g blueberries (35 calories)
1 slice of lean ham (40g, 50 calories)

Dinner *358 calories with rice; 218 without*
Chickpea curry: heat a pan and spray with oil (10 calories),
fry ½ a chopped onion (75g, 27 calories) and a crushed clove
of garlic (3 calories) for 2 mins or until softened. Add 1 tsp
curry powder and a pinch of chilli flakes (or more, to taste)
and cook for a further 2 mins. Add 100ml boiling water, ½
veggie stock cube (10 calories), 1 tbsp tomato purée (14
calories) and ½ a tin of chickpeas (120g drained weight, 132
calories). Simmer for 5-10 mins, add 5-6 cherry tomatoes
(75g, 14 calories) and a handful of spinach leaves (30g, 8
calories) towards the end of cooking time. Season and serve
with brown basmati rice (115g cooked rice, 140 calories)

Daily total: 505 calories

DAY 10

Breakfast *240 calories*
Grilled kipper (100g, 240 calories)

Dinner *256 calories*
Fast Day insalata Caprese: slice 3 balls of low-fat mozzarella
(110g, 185 calories) and place on a plate with 2 sliced beef
tomatoes (200g, 36 calories). Scatter with fresh basil and
drizzle with 1 tsp good-quality balsamic vinegar (5 calories)

8 strawberries (30 calories)

Daily total: 496 calories

FAST 600 MENU PLANS FOR MEN

DAY 1

Breakfast *270 calories*
Mushroom and spinach frittata: fry ½ a small sliced onion
(75g, 27 calories) in 1 tsp olive oil (40 calories). Add 4 small
chopped mushrooms (20g, 3 calories). Cook until tender. Add
a generous handful of spinach (30g, 8 calories); cook for 2
mins. Pour over 2 beaten eggs (170 calories). Season and
cook for 5 mins, and finish under a hot grill until eggs are just
set.

25 raspberries (100g, 22 calories)

Dinner *333 calories*
Seared tuna: heat a griddle pan and sear a seasoned tuna
steak (160g, 225 calories) on both sides using no fat, but
squeezing in lemon if necessary. Cut 1 red pepper (160g, 50
calories) and ½ medium courgette (80g, 18 calories) into long
strips. Mix in a bowl with 1 tsp olive oil (40 calories), season,
and grill on medium-high heat for 5 mins each side. Dress
with a squeeze of lemon

Daily total: 603 calories

DAY 2

Breakfast *198 calories*
2 large poached eggs (180 calories) with 1 grilled tomato
(100g, 18 calories)

Dinner *402 calories*
Pesto salmon: preheat oven to 180°C. Smear a salmon fillet
(150g, 275 calories) with 2 tsp pesto (52 calories). Season
and bake until fish is cooked through, approximately 15 mins.
Serve with baked veggies – ½ a medium courgette, cut into
ribbons (80g, 18 calories), 10 tomatoes on the vine (140g,
27 calories) and ½ a red pepper (80g, 25 calories), cut into
strips; spray with a little oil (5 calories) and place in hot oven
for 6-8 mins, turning halfway through.

Daily total: 600 calories

DAY 3

Breakfast *317 calories*
<u>Spiced pear porridge:</u> simmer 30g jumbo oats (114 calories), 250ml skimmed milk (105 calories) and ½ a peeled and diced pear (90g, 47 calories), with ½ tsp cinnamon and a grate of nutmeg. Stir and cook until porridge is thickened to your liking. Serve with 5 roughly chopped hazelnuts (37 calories), adding 1 tsp agave nectar to taste (14 calories).

Dinner *295 calories*
<u>No-carb Caesar salad:</u> grill 2 slices of Parma ham (50g, 76 calories) for 4-5 mins, turning once, until crispy.
Slice 1 chicken breast (100g, 148 calories) into two. Grill for about 5-8 mins each side, or until cooked. Cut into pieces and place on a substantial bed of chopped Cos lettuce (100g, 16 calories). Serve with 1 tbsp grated Parmesan (45 calories), and 1 tbsp reduced-calorie Caesar salad dressing (15g, 10 calories – eg Sainsbury's Be Good To Yourself). Crumble the grilled Parma ham over the top

Daily total: 612 calories

DAY 4

Breakfast *290 calories*
Grilled kipper (100g, 240 calories)
2 tangerines (160g, 50 calories)

Dinner *317 calories*
<u>Marinated steak with Asian coleslaw:</u> marinate a piece of sirloin steak (130g, 170 calories) in a mixture of soy, the juice of 1 lime and a crushed garlic clove (3 calories). Grill until cooked to your liking, turning once and set aside to rest. Combine 1 grated carrot (80g, 28 calories) with 90g Savoy cabbage cut into thin strips (24 calories), and a handful of coriander (2 calories). For dressing, mix 1 tsp sugar (16 calories) with 1 tbsp Thai fish sauce (10 calories), the juice of half a lime (1 calorie), and a crushed clove of garlic (3 calories). Pour over salad and top with 10g chopped roasted, unsalted peanuts (60 calories) and thin slices of rested steak.

Daily total: 607 calories

DAY 5

Breakfast *219 calories*
English breakfast: grill 2 lean rashers of bacon (50g, 115 calories), 1 small sausage (20g, 59 calories), 10 large cherry tomatoes on the vine (140g, 27 calories) and 1 seasoned Portobello mushroom (70g, 10 calories) to your liking and serve with a generous handful of spinach (30g, 8 calories), wilted for 2 mins in a pan with a dash of boiling water. Dry spinach thoroughly and season well with sea salt and black pepper

Dinner *384 calories*
Roast mackerel and vegetables: place a mackerel fillet (150g, 320 calories) on top of 2 sliced tomatoes (170g, 30 calories). Wrap in foil and roast in a hot oven for 10–15 mins or until fish is done. Serve with a big pile of tenderstem broccoli (100g, 33 calories), seasoned and dressed with the juice of ½ a lemon (1 calorie)

Daily total: 603 calories

DAY 6

Breakfast *298 calories*
1 small pot of fat-free natural yoghurt (150g, 62 calories)
1 chopped banana (100g, 95 calories)
6 strawberries (72g, 20 calories)
100g blueberries (70 calories)
10 almonds, chopped (9g, 51 calories)

Dinner *314 calories*
<u>Cumin-turkey burgers with corn on the cob:</u> combine 125g
turkey mince (123 calories), 1 finely chopped spring onion,
1 tbsp beaten egg (35 calories), ½ finely chopped red chilli
(1 calorie), 1 clove crushed garlic (3 calories), ½ tsp ground
cumin, ½ tsp ground coriander and salt and pepper. Leave
to marinate for half an hour in the fridge. Shape into 2 patties
and grill for 5-7 mins on each side, or until cooked through.
Serve with lemon-dressed salad leaves (20 calories) and
small corn on the cob, boiled and dusted with paprika (132
calories)

Daily total: 612 calories

DAY 7

Breakfast *261 calories*
Scrambled eggs: add 1 tbsp skimmed milk (5 calories) to 2
large beaten eggs (180 calories) and scramble in a non-stick
pan. Serve with 2 slices of Parma ham (50g, 76 calories)

Dinner *332 calories*
Spiced dhal with naan: in 1 tsp olive oil (40 calories), fry
½ a finely chopped onion (75g, 27 calories), 1 clove of
crushed garlic (3 calories) and 1 tsp finely chopped ginger (3
calories). Cook for 5 mins. Add half a pint (280ml) of water,
50g washed, drained red lentils (159 calories), a pinch each
of cumin, coriander, turmeric and cayenne pepper. Boil for 20
mins or until lentils are tender. Season with salt and pepper,
and garnish with 2 tbsp low-fat natural yoghurt (30 calories)
and a handful of torn coriander leaves. Serve with half a low-
fat naan bread (70 calories)

Daily total: 593 calories

DAY 8

Breakfast *237 calories*
2 large boiled eggs (180 calories)
5 asparagus spears (125g, 33 calories), to dip
1 plum (24 calories)

Dinner *365 calories*
Thai steak salad: grill a sirloin steak (140g, 188 calories)
on both sides until cooked to your liking, rest well and slice
very thinly. Serve on a pile of shredded lettuce (100g, 14
calories), and shredded Savoy cabbage (100g, 24 calories),
beansprouts (50g, 17 calories) and 1 large shredded carrot
(130g, 51 calories), dressed with: juice of 1 lime (1 calorie), 1
tsp sugar (16 calories), a crushed clove of garlic (3 calories),
a chopped, deseeded chilli (1 calorie), 1 tsp sesame oil (40
calories) and 1 tbsp Thai fish sauce (10 calories)

Daily total: 602 calories

DAY 9

Breakfast *205 calories*
1 small pot of fat-free natural yoghurt (150g, 62 calories)
1 small chopped banana (100g, 95 calories)
1 tbsp sugar-free muesli, not granola, stirred through (15g, 48 calories)

Dinner *383 calories*
Roast pork: serve 150g lean roast pork loin (289 calories) with steamed cauliflower (60g, 17 calories) and broccoli (50g, 17 calories). Drizzle with 1 tbsp meat juices (60 calories)

Daily total: 588 calories

DAY 10

Breakfast *172 calories*
Smoked salmon (90g, 170 calories)
Lemon wedges and chopped chives to serve (2 calories)

Dinner *426 calories*
Bacon & butterbean soup: fry 2 rashers of lean bacon (54g, 116 calories) in 1 tsp olive oil (40 calories) for 2 mins. Add 30g finely chopped onion (10 calories), ½ a chopped leek (50g, 7 calories), 40g sliced carrot (14 calories), and ½ diced stalk of celery (4 calories). Cook for 5 mins, adding a splash of water if it sticks. Add butterbeans (200g, 210 calories), half a pint of water (280ml) and ½ a vegetable stock cube (10 calories). Simmer for 20 mins. Season. Blend until desired consistency, or simply mash for chunkier texture

4 strawberries (50g, 15 calories)

Daily total: 598 calories

THE FAST DIET'S GREATEST HITS

Over the past two years, some recipes from the Fast Diet cookbooks have emerged as firm favourites – chiefly because they are quick, easy, tasty and surprisingly low in calories, while still packed full of flavour. Here, then, are our top ten dishes to include in your 5:2 repertoire; note that some are best cooked for two or four people, so the calories listed here are *per portion*.

<u>Spiced chicken with warm lentils and roasted garlic</u>

399 calories per portion
Serves 4

For the marinade
3cm fresh root ginger, grated
1 tsp ground coriander
1 tsp ground cumin
1 tsp paprika
1 tsp ground turmeric
Juice of a lemon
2 tsp olive oil
Salt and pepper

1 medium chicken (approximately 1.5kg)
1 head of garlic, sliced in half across the equator
125g Puy lentils, washed
2 tbsp water
Generous handful of parsley, chopped

Generous handful of coriander, chopped
1 tbsp chives, snipped
Juice of half a lemon
Salt and pepper

Whisk marinade ingredients and rub into chicken, working under the skin. Refrigerate for an hour, or overnight if possible. Preheat oven to 180°C. Place chicken and garlic in a roasting pan and roast for an hour and 10 mins – or until the juices run clear. Remove garlic and chicken from oven and rest on a separate plate, retaining the juices in the pan. While the chicken is cooking, place lentils in a saucepan, cover with water and bring to the boil; when cooked but still al dente, drain and refresh with cold water, drain again and add them to the roasting pan along with 2 tbsp water. Heat through, scraping the pan for sticky bits on the base. Remove from heat and add chopped herbs and lemon juice. Stir well, season and serve with the torn chicken (skin removed) and soft garlic.

Goan aubergine curry

173 calories per portion (250 with basmati rice)
Serves 2

1 tsp cumin seeds, dry-fried and ground
2 tsp coriander seeds, dry-fried and ground
½ tsp cayenne pepper
½ tsp ground turmeric
1 green chilli, deseeded and finely sliced
2 garlic cloves, crushed
3cm fresh root ginger, grated
200ml water
300ml half-fat coconut milk
1 tbsp tamarind paste
1 large aubergine, cut lengthways into 5mm slices
Salt and pepper

Place ground roasted cumin and coriander seeds in a large saucepan along with the cayenne, turmeric, chilli, garlic, ginger and add the water. Bring to a simmer, then add the coconut milk and tamarind paste. Cook on a low heat stirring occasionally, until the sauce has slightly thickened – around 10 mins. Heat grill to medium-high. Place aubergine slices on a foil-lined baking tray and brush with a little of the curried sauce. Grill until they are soft and cooked through, turning once and brushing the other side with the sauce – about 10-15 minutes in total. Arrange the aubergine in a serving dish, and spoon over the rest of the hot curry sauce. Serve with 50g brown basmati rice per person.

Vietnamese prawn pho

48 calories per portion
(add 10-15 calories for every 50g of additional veg)
Serves 4

2 lemongrass stems, outer leaves removed, inner stem
   finely chopped
2 tsp fresh root ginger, grated
4 kaffir lime leaves, torn
1.5l vegetable or fish stock
1 tsp palm, or or light soft brown, sugar
3 tbsp Thai fish sauce
Juice of a lime
10 large prawns, shelled and deveined
50g bean sprouts
Fresh Thai basil leaves, mint, coriander and sliced red
   chilli to serve

Use a pestle and mortar to grind lemongrass, ginger and
kaffir lime leaves. Add paste to a large saucepan with stock
and boil for 10 mins. Add sugar, fish sauce and lime juice,
tasting to check for balance. Cook prawns in broth till
pink – about 2-3 mins. Add beansprouts, plenty of herbs
and red chilli to serve.

Skinny spag bol

180 calories per portion
Serves 4

Cooking oil spray
400g lean minced beef
1 large onion, diced
1 garlic clove, crushed
1 celery stick, diced
1 red pepper, diced
200g mushrooms, chopped
½ tsp mixed herbs
1 tsp mixed spice
1 400g tin cherry tomatoes
3 tbsp tomato purée
1 courgette, diced
200ml beef stock (or boiling water plus an Oxo cube)
1 tsp Marmite
Salt and pepper

Spray a large pan with a little oil, fry the meat until it is browned and then set aside. Add onion, garlic, celery and pepper to the pan and cook gently for 2-3 mins, or until softened. Add mushrooms, herbs, mixed spice, tomatoes and tomato purée and cook for a further 3 mins. Add browned mince and courgette, together with the stock and Marmite. Cover and simmer, stirring occasionally, for 30 minutes – longer if possible, to enrich the sauce. Check seasoning and serve.

Instead of pasta, serve with…

- steamed broccoli and cauliflower florets (+ 35 calories per 100g)
- veg 'noodles' – stir-fried ribbons of courgette, carrot and leek (+ 35 calories per 100g)

Huevos rancheros

283 calories per portion
Serves 1

1 tsp olive oil
2 spring onions, finely chopped
1 red pepper, sliced
¼ tsp chilli flakes
1 200g tin chopped tomatoes
1 tsp balsamic vinegar
2 medium eggs
Handful of flat-leaf parsley, roughly chopped
Salt and pepper

Heat oil in a small frying pan and gently fry spring onion, red pepper and chilli flakes for 3 mins. Add tomatoes and vinegar. Season, stir and simmer for 5 mins. Make two dips in the sauce and crack an egg into each. Continue cooking until whites have begun to set, then cover the pan and cook until they are completely set, but the yolks are still runny. Sprinkle with parsley and serve.

Super-fast Thai green chicken curry

331 calories per portion
Serves 2

400ml half-fat coconut milk
1 tbsp Thai green curry paste
100ml chicken stock
1 tbsp lime juice
1 tbsp Thai fish sauce
200g chicken breast, cut into strips
200g vegetables; choose a mix from baby 'pea'
  aubergines, young courgette, baby sweetcorn, mange
  tout, broccoli florets, pak choi, thinly sliced peppers,
  green beans, shiitake or oyster mushrooms, bean
  sprouts, frozen petits pois or spinach
1 green chilli, finely sliced
Handful of coriander leaves
Lime wedges, to serve

Heat 1 tbsp of coconut milk in a pan, stir in the curry
paste and cook for 2 mins to release its flavour. Add the
rest of the coconut milk, stock, lime juice and fish sauce.
Bring to a low simmer and cook for 10 mins. Add the
chicken strips and vegetables of your choice, and continue
to simmer until chicken is cooked through – about 5
mins. Top with fresh chilli and coriander leaves, and serve
with a wedge of lime.

Prawn and asparagus stir-fry

105 calories per portion
Serves 2

1 tsp vegetable oil
1 medium onion, sliced
2 garlic cloves, crushed
1 tsp ground ginger
1 red bird's eye chilli, deseeded and finely chopped
4 spring onions, finely sliced on the diagonal
1 lemongrass stem, bruised
2 lime leaves
3 tbsp Thai fish sauce
2 tbsp boiling water
½ tsp palm sugar
12 raw king prawns
300g asparagus, halved lengthways and cut into 3cm pieces
Coriander, Thai basil leaves, lime wedges to serve

Heat the oil in a wok, and stir-fry onion, garlic, ginger and chilli until softened. Add spring onion, cook for a further minute, then add then add lemongrass, lime leaves, fish sauce, water and sugar. Stir, then add the prawns and asparagus. Cook on a high heat for 3 mins or until the prawns are pink and the asparagus is al dente. Remove lemongrass. Serve with fresh coriander leaves, Thai basil and a wedge of lime.

Red lentil tikka masala

218 calories per portion
Serves 4

For the masala paste
2 tsp garam masala
2 tsp chilli flakes
2 tsp smoked paprika
1 tsp cumin seeds, dry-fried and ground
1 tsp coriander seeds, dry-fried and ground
2cm fresh root ginger, grated
1 tbsp groundnut oil
2 tbsp tomato purée
Salt and pepper
Handful of fresh coriander

For the curry
1½ tbsp vegetable oil
1 red onion, diced
2 tbsp masala paste
1 garlic clove, crushed
1 400g tin chopped tomatoes
250ml vegetable stock
200g red lentils, rinsed
200g young spinach leaves, washed
2 tbsp low-fat natural yoghurt

Pulse paste ingredients in a processor. Heat the oil in a large frying pan, add onion and cook until softened, around 3-4 mins. Add garlic and cook for a further minute. Stir in the masala paste and cook for a couple of mins to release the flavours, then add tomatoes and vegetable stock and bring to the boil. Add lentils, reduce heat and simmer for 20 mins. Remove from heat and add spinach leaves, allowing them to wilt in the warmth. If necessary, loosen the mixture with a little more hot stock. Serve with the yoghurt spooned over.

Madras beef with a tomato and red onion salad

319 calories per portion
Serves 4

1 tbsp vegetable oil
1 onion, sliced
2 garlic cloves, crushed
2 green peppers, deseeded and sliced
3 cardamom pods, bruised
1 cinnamon stick
4 red chillies, 2 deseeded and finely chopped,
  2 split lengthways
2 tsp Madras curry powder (or more to taste)
1 400g tin cherry tomatoes, chopped
1 tbsp tomato purée
800g stewing or braising steak, trimmed of fat and cubed
½ tsp caster sugar
Salt and pepper
450ml beef stock (or boiling water plus an Oxo cube)
¼ red onion, 1 ripe tomato, fresh coriander, to serve

Preheat oven to 170°C. Heat oil in a flameproof casserole dish and fry onion, garlic, green peppers, cardamom, cinnamon stick and chopped chilli for 5-7 mins. Add curry powder, stir, cook for a further minute or two and add chopped tomatoes and purée. Cook over a medium heat for 5 mins, stirring. Add beef, halved chillies, sugar, salt and pepper, stirring to ensure the meat gets a good coating and cook for a further 2 mins. Add stock, bring to a simmer, cover and transfer to the oven. Cook for 1½ hours or until beef is tender. Serve with a salad of thinly sliced red onion and ripe tomatoes, with torn coriander and plenty of black pepper.

Field mushrooms with mozzarella, pecorino and spinach

159 calories per portion
Serves 1

100g baby spinach leaves, washed and wilted
½ tsp chilli flakes
1 garlic clove, crushed
1 large or 2 medium field mushrooms, washed and dried
50g low-fat mozzarella, torn
2 tsp pecorino, grated or shaved
Fresh thyme leaves
Salt and pepper
Salad leaves, to serve

Preheat grill to 200°C. Mix the spinach, chilli flakes and garlic in a small bowl. Fill the mushroom cap with the mixture, sprinkle over the mozzarella, pecorino and thyme leaves, season and grill for 7-10 mins, or until cheese has melted, and mushroom is cooked but still firm. Serve with dressed salad leaves.

AND SIX TASTY NEW RECIPES TO TRY...

Dijon chicken dippers with peas

281 calories per portion
Serves 2

1 tbsp Dijon mustard
2 tbsp low-fat natural yoghurt
1 tsp herbes de Provence
Salt and pepper
300g mini chicken breast fillets
200g frozen peas
6 mint leaves, finely chopped
½ red chilli, deseeded and finely chopped
1 tsp butter

In a small bowl, combine Dijon, yoghurt and herbs. Season and add chicken pieces, stirring so they are well coated. Refrigerate until needed (up to 24 hours). Heat grill or griddle pan and cook marinated chicken pieces until done (8-10 minutes). Boil the peas and put half aside. Mash the remaining half with a fork, stir in the whole peas, along with the mint, chilli and butter. Stir, season well and serve alongside the chicken.

Masala salmon with spiced spinach

398 calories per portion
Serves 2

100g low-fat natural yoghurt
1 tbsp masala paste
1 tsp cumin seeds
Salt and pepper
2 salmon fillets (approx. 100g each)

For the spiced spinach
Cooking oil spray
2 spring onions, sliced
1 garlic clove, crushed
½ tsp ground coriander
Pinch cayenne pepper (to taste)
½ tsp garam masala
2 cardamom pods, bruised
300g spinach leaves, washed
Salt and pepper
A squeeze of lemon

Preheat the oven to 180°C. In a small bowl, combine yoghurt, masala paste and cumin seeds, season, then add the salmon fillets and coat well. Bake the salmon until opaque (approx. 15 mins). Meanwhile, heat a pan and spray with oil. Sauté spring onion, garlic and spices gently for 3-4 minutes, or until softened. Add spinach, allowing it to wilt down in the heat and adding a dash of water if necessary to prevent it sticking. Cook for 3-4 minutes, stirring gently. Remove from heat, season and add a squeeze of lemon. Serve alongside the warm baked salmon.

My Thai mussels

470 calories per portion
Serves 2

2cm fresh root ginger, peeled and julienned
1 lemongrass stalk, finely sliced
1 kaffir lime leaf
1 red chilli, deseeded and finely sliced (to taste)
1 400ml tin half-fat coconut milk
1 tbsp Thai fish sauce
1 tsp sesame oil
1kg mussels, washed and debearded – discard any that aren't tightly closed
Juice of half a lime
Handful of fresh coriander leaves
1 spring onion, finely sliced
Lime wedges and red chilli to serve

Place the ginger, lemongrass, lime leaf and chilli in a large pan with the coconut milk, fish sauce and sesame oil. Bring to the boil and simmer for 5-10 mins. Add the mussels and cover the pan. Cook for 5 minutes, shaking the pan occasionally, until the mussels are open and cooked (discard any that are shut). Add lime juice, then serve in a large bowl, garnished with coriander leaves, spring onion, lime wedges and a little more red chilli, if desired.

Warm aubergine salad with chickpeas and Halloumi

471 calories per portion
Serves 2

1 tbsp olive oil
1 tsp ground cumin
1 tsp paprika
Salt and pepper
1-2 aubergines (approx. 400g), sliced into pound-coin
  widths
150g reduced-fat Halloumi cheese, sliced
1 400g tin chickpeas, rinsed and drained
200g cherry tomatoes, halved
Handful of flat-leaf parsley leaves, chopped

For the dressing
Handful of mint leaves, finely chopped
100g low-fat natural yoghurt
1 garlic clove, crushed
2 tsp lemon juice
Pinch of salt

Combine dressing ingredients. In a separate small bowl, mix olive oil, cumin, paprika, salt and pepper and brush onto both sides of aubergine slices. Heat griddle pan and cook slices, turning once, until golden (approx. 5 minutes on each side) – then set aside. Using the same pan, cook the Halloumi slices, turning them once, until they are lightly coloured. Combine chickpeas, tomatoes and parsley with 2 tsp of the dressing. Top with cooked aubergine and Halloumi slices, drizzle with the remaining dressing and add a final twist of pepper.

Baked butternut with courgette and tomato

248 calories per portion, 290 with feta
Serves 2

3-4 young/medium courgettes, sliced on the diagonal into pound-coin widths
400g butternut squash, peeled and cubed
1 vine of cherry tomatoes
6 black olives (optional)
One head of garlic, halved around the equator
Half a lemon
2 tbsp olive oil
Handful of fresh thyme leaves
Salt and pepper

Preheat oven to 180°C. Place the prepared veggies in a small ovenproof dish, add olive oil and juice of half a lemon, along with the lemon husk. Season well. Bake for 25 mins until garlic is softened and the veggies are beginning to caramelise. Perhaps serve with a sprinkle of feta (25g per portion; add 42 calories). Alternatively, this works well as a side dish with any roast or grilled meat.

Butterbean and chorizo hotpot

249 calories per portion
Serves 2

30g chorizo, finely chopped
1 medium onion, peeled and finely diced
2 garlic cloves, peeled and crushed
1 400g tin butter beans, rinsed and drained
1 400g tin chopped tomatoes
1 tbsp tomato purée
1 tsp smoked paprika
Pinch of sugar
2 tbsp water
Salt and pepper
Handful parsley, roughly chopped, to serve

Heat a medium-sized pan and gently fry the chorizo to release its colour and flavour. Add onion and garlic, and cook them gently until they have softened (approx. 5 minutes). Add butterbeans, tomatoes, tomato purée, paprika and sugar. Simmer for 15 mins, stirring occasionally. Add 2 tbsp water, or a little more if the pan starts to look dry. Season and serve.

STRAIGHT TO THE PLATE

I included some of these 'fridge and cupboard' ideas in *Fast Cook*, and they proved a popular way to get through supper on a Fast Day with minimum fuss. Not recipes so much as great flavour combinations, these trios can be grabbed from your fridge and kitchen cupboards, on days when you just don't want to think too hard about food. Use lemon juice or balsamic vinegar (I like it in spray form) where necessary. Then just add a plate and a fork.

- Shredded white cabbage + sliced red onion + hard-boiled egg (1 medium) **120 calories**

- Smoked salmon (50g) + hard-boiled egg (1 medium) + sliced fennel **180 calories**

- Broad beans (100g) + radicchio + pecorino (30g) **196 calories**

- Lean roast beef (100g) + horseradish crème fraîche (1 tbsp) + little gem lettuce **203 calories**

- Chicken tikka pieces (130g) + sliced beef tomato + cucumber raita (2 tbsp) **216 calories**

- Avocado (half) + prawns (50g) + low-fat crème fraîche (1 tbsp) **221 calories**

- Parma ham (4 slices) + melon (1 slice) + 8 strawberries **228 calories**

- Mozzarella (50g) + avocado (half) + 2 ripe tomatoes **238 calories**

- Baby spinach + Parma ham (4 slices) + shaved Parmesan (30g) **224 calories**

- Low-fat hummus (100g) + raw veggies (200g) + jalapeños **246 calories**

- Tinned tuna (120g) + cannellini beans (125g) + red onion **268 calories**

- Cooked turkey breast (200g) + rocket + pine nuts (10g) **269 calories**

- Smoked chicken (150g) + romaine lettuce + cashews (20g) **276 calories**

- Blanched French beans + cooked king prawns (140g) + low-fat feta (100g) **289 calories**

- Roast beetroot (100g) + low-fat Halloumi 100g + rocket **293 calories**

- Low-fat feta (100g) + hard-boiled egg (1 medium) + quarter of a red cabbage **285 calories**

- Pilchards in olive oil (100g) + 10 cherry tomatoes + steamed broccoli florets **323 calories**

- Smoked mackerel (150g) + watercress + 4 plum tomatoes **354 calories**

- Beef carpaccio (150g) + toasted pine nuts (10g) + rocket + Parmesan (30g) **404 calories**

FAST DAY SNACKS

As we all know, there's little point in grazing on a Fast Day – it would soon eliminate the point of the exercise. But some people need a little lift, particularly in the early days when their appetite is adjusting to the new regime. It's best to avoid easy carbs and go instead for fresh, raw ingredients. Have them prepped and handy in the fridge. Nuts, though high in calories, are full of protein and good fats, and just a few will help you feel full.

- Liquorice root to chew **0 calories**
- Harley's sugar-free jelly pots **4 calories**
- 60g cherries **33 calories**
- 100g blackberries **25 calories**
- Fresh strawberries **30 calories for 8-10**
- A miso soup sachet, or a cup of hot Bovril **32 calories**
- Crudités: carrot sticks, celery stalks, cucumber sticks, raw pepper, watercress, radishes, cherry tomatoes **approx 20 calories per serving**
- A tbsp cottage cheese **20 calories**
- 1 apple, sliced, including skin and core – add a squeeze of lemon juice **60 calories**
- A hard-boiled egg **75-90 calories** (depending on size)
- 1 tbsp hummus **28 calories**

- A handful of frozen grapes **60 calories**

- Pistachios **60 calories for 10**

- Almonds **80 calories for 6**

- Plain edamame – 60g, steamed and served warm with a little rock salt **84 calories**

- 25g Edam **80 calories**

- A couple of hard-boiled quail's eggs **90 calories**

- 1 tbsp pumpkin and sunflower seeds **90 calories**

- 25g air-popped popcorn **148 calories**

THE 5:2 SHOPPING LIST

Get in the habit of having Fast-friendly food around – just enough to allow you to grab a quick meal when you're fasting and famished. Here's what you might have to hand...

In the fridge
Eggs

Half-fat hummus, low-fat natural yoghurt, half-fat crème fraîche

Feta, cottage cheese and low-fat mozzarella

Spring onions

Chillies

Fresh herbs

Non-starchy veggies: cauliflower, broccoli, peppers, radishes, cherry tomatoes, celery, cucumber, mushrooms, lettuce, sugar snaps, mange touts, salad leaves and a bag of young spinach

Carrots

Lemons

Strawberries, blueberries, apples

In the larder
Tinned tuna in spring water

Tins of beans – cannellini, borlotti, flageolet – and chickpeas

Tins of tomatoes

Tomato purée

Garlic

Onions – red and white

Mustard – Dijon and English

Vinegar – balsamic and white wine; try balsamic spritzer on salad

Olive oil

Cooking oil spray

Spices, including cumin and coriander

Chilli flakes

Nuts – unsalted are preferable; eat with caution as they are generally high in calories

Pickles – guindillas, jalapeños, cornichons, capers

Marmite, Oxo cubes, stock cubes, miso paste

Sea salt & freshly ground black pepper

No-sugar Alpen

No-sugar jelly

Shirataki noodles

Miso-soup sachets

In the freezer

Root ginger – it is best grated from frozen

Stock, in empty (clean) soup and milk cartons

Soup – home-made or shop bought, in single portions

Blueberries, a cool little snack (strawberries do not freeze well)

Peas

CHOOSING THE RIGHT READY-MEAL

If a ready-meal is your only salvation during a busy week on the Fast Diet, then here are a few tips to help you make the right choices.

- Look for meals with plants at their heart — accompanied by some 'good' protein and slow-burn carbs. Avoid pre-cooked pasta and potato dishes

- Check the portion size. Don't finish the box just because it tells you to. One Fast Dieter says she regularly uses a 'Serves 2' meal to feed three

- Supplement your ready meal with easy-access fresh vits: grab half a bag of spinach leaves, a handful of rocket, little gem lettuce — whatever it takes to get your greens

- A chiller-cabinet soup can be a good option: again, look at the serving size and the calorie count

- Even if you're eating in a hurry, try to do it sitting down, giving food your full attention

Reasonable examples of Fast-friendly ready-meals widely available in the UK might include:

- Sainsbury's My Goodness! Tom Yum King Prawn Noodle Soup **263 calories**

- Sainsbury's My Goodness! Red Thai Vegetable Curry **361 calories**

- Pret a Manger Salmon and Quinoa Protein Pot **145 calories**

- Pret a Manger Tuna Nicoise Salad **168 calories**

- Tesco Healthy Living Chicken with Whole Grains **361 calories**

- Waitrose Kirsty's Moroccan Vegetables with Quinoa **276 calories**

THE FAST DIET AND ME

Testimonials & Tweets

Mark Lovell, aged 44, Germany
Lost 2st 6lb (15.4kg) in 4 months

'I never thought I would be writing a piece on dieting in any capacity. However, this comes from the heart as a very satisfied Fast Diet convert.

'In July 2013, after a dream vacation in the States, I topped the scales at an all-time high of 18 stone and could not ignore the fact that I was overweight, despite claims that I supposedly "carried it well".

'Looking back now, something must have gone "click" in my mind after watching Dr Michael Mosley's excellent documentary, and I decided to take action. I was ready to try something different.

'I plumped for Mondays and Thursdays as my fasting days and soon noticed a change in my habits. I learned that 600 calories is actually quite manageable with LOTS of salad and vegetables and that this is not a punishing diet. I lost nearly two and a half stone in four months and have been stable for more than 14 months. I learned that I didn't need to eat all the time and that in fact I could go a long time without eating. The beauty of the Fast Diet for me is that I can still eat what I want on those non-fasting days. My favourite meal is still an Indian curry.

'The biggest motivation is that the scales do not lie – this works. The Fast Diet has now become a way of life, I am not fighting food any more and I am enjoying life to the full. And not only do I feel hyper-energised, people have even told me I look a tad younger!'

Mo Hayter, aged 66, Hampshire
Lost 1st 10lb (11kg) in 6 months

'I started my Fast Diet on 21 January this year when I read about it in the *Mail on Sunday*. I was about 3st over-weight with a BMI of 31 and all my attempts at losing weight had failed. I was really concerned on the first day that I'd faint or have some adverse effects, but I was fine and so I persevered. I lost 16lb in the first two months, after which the rate of my weight loss slowed down a lot but it is now steady. I've lost a total of 24lb and my BMI is down to 27. It's a way of life for me now so I intend to continue!

'Before I started the diet, my blood pressure was very high, but it has been reduced significantly and I'm sure that's down to losing so much weight. My cholesterol was also very high, particularly the LDL (low-density lipoprotein), so I can't wait to see if it's improved (as Dr Mosley's did) at my next check-up. One thing's for sure, I feel so much healthier and so happy that I've found such an easy way of losing weight. Not to mention my asthma has also improved.'

Stella Minnet, aged 60, Swindon
Lost 3st (19kg) in 1 year

'When I started the Fast Diet 12 months ago, I weighed nearly 12 and a half stone, the heaviest I had ever been. Even though I had been doing up to two or three exercise classes a week for the past three years, I'd steadily been putting on weight. I'm now down to 9st 5lb, a loss of three stone. I weigh less than I did when I got married at age 20! I love this way of life and am proud to have encouraged others to follow it too with great success. I still do several classes of exercises a week including body pump, circuits and have started running again, which is so much easier at this weight! I'm now in size 12 jeans, down from a 16 this time last year.

'The biggest change is the way I feel – being lighter on

my feet, wearing smaller clothes and taking pride in my achievement. And I really enjoy all the compliments!'

Monica Michael, aged 27, Cyprus
Lost 2st 8lb (17.7kg) in 5 months

'I am a sufferer of PCOS (polycystic ovary syndrome) and the Fast Diet has been AMAZING for me. I started it a little over 5 months ago and have already lost two and a half stone. I have also cured my insulin resistance and no longer need medication for it, and am no longer pre-diabetic. My PCOS is under control and my sugar levels have stabilised. My energy levels have soared and I eat a lot more healthily now as I really think before I eat instead of just stuffing my face with processed junk foods. Buying *The Fast Beach Diet* book was one of the best things I have ever done.

'I'm so glad I took the challenge to lose my last kilos before my holiday in Crete this year. I'm in better shape now than even before I had my three boys and am happy to wear my bikini for the first time in years!'

Stephen Morris, aged 44, Exmoor
Lost 3st (19kg) in 3 months

'Over the years I have tried just about every diet going

but have never really been able to stick with anything for more than 10 days at a time. I'd get fed up when I woke up each morning, knowing that I faced yet another day of going without enjoyable food. To me, the word "diet" is really another word for "deprivation".

'This is why the 5:2 has been such a revelation to me. I started doing the Fast Diet around three months ago. The first Fast Day wasn't easy, but then again it wasn't as hard as I expected either. The second Fast Day was similar. After a week I'd dropped 5lb and I was happy. By the fourth week, the odd person began to notice a change, which was a great boost. All of a sudden the fasts were becoming quite easy, I was used to them. In a strange way I started to look forward to them. I felt inspired and I was noticing things beyond the scales – an inch lost just about everywhere. One month became two and people really started to comment on my changing appearance. Suddenly it crept up on me, I'd been doing this for three months and had lost 3st; all without really having to try too hard. This is so easy compared to anything else I've attempted. It really is a great way of eating as I still have a social life. A couple of days a week of discipline against five days of not worrying seems a very good deal to me.

'So what's worth noting? Before starting the diet, I had a diabetes test and my levels were very high. My test a couple of weeks back showed that I no longer have anything to worry about. Energy-wise, I feel better than I have in years, no longer dreading exercise but enjoying it. I've walked the local cliff path where I live for years and I'm literally doing it in half the time it used to take me. Also, after years of terrible insomnia I'm starting to sleep better. I awake refreshed in the morning. Everyone notices the changes now! I'm getting into clothes I've not worn for years. On my non-Fast Days, I can go out and eat and drink what I want without guilt. But if I have a really heavy weekend I'll sometimes do an extra fast to compensate, but not always. I have just one rule: never ever quit a Fast Day. What keeps me going is knowing that tomorrow I can eat normally again.

'Oh, and one other thing, I used to be totally dependent on sugar – not any more. I can take it or leave it. If you'd said that to me three months ago, I'd have just laughed!'

Debi Clayton, aged 49, Northants
Lost 3st 5lb (22.4kg) in 6 months

'I downloaded *The Fast Diet* at the start of the New Year (2014) because I hated how miserable my weight was making me. I rarely went out other than to go to work (I'm a secondary school teacher) and blamed the menopause for my considerable and rapid weight gain. I was making excuses in order not to walk our dogs so my husband did it because I got so tired, yet I was drinking a glass of wine most evenings to help me relax and fall asleep. Apart from HRT patches for the menopause, I was not on any other medication and I ate healthy food – or thought I did. The fact is that it became unhealthy due to the amount I was eating. I had no portion control. My porridge oats breakfast with water, yoghurt and berries was clocking up 700 calories!

'After reading Michael and Mimi's book, I was convinced that I could manage the restricted calorie intake just twice a week. I was most impressed with the information about hunger not growing or worsening as time passed. I was very afraid of hunger!

'I started on 13 January: my Fast Day consisted of black coffee (easy), sparkling mineral water with fresh lemon slices, two hard-boiled eggs and a pear, all consumed at lunchtime; then chicken salad and Diet Coke for dinner.

'I was hungry but the pangs did not amount to more than a discomfort which I soon found could be pacified with fluid and staying busy. The weight doesn't drop off in crazy amounts. Most weeks I lose between half a pound and 2lb but I've had fortnights of no loss, and then other weeks when I've lost 2½lb.

'I am now jogging with my younger dog! I can jump out of bed and go for a 6am run, I do my Zumba lessons, often with ankle weights and intensity level 3, I never consume wine to help me sleep. Actually, these days, I sleep like a baby regardless of my calorie intake. I feel alive and in charge of my life. I will not stop fasting just because I am a healthy weight. The benefits of feeling clear-headed, energised and enjoying food tastes and textures is something I can't give up. I have played about with my fasting methods and now on a Fast Day prefer to consume fluids and save my calorie allowance in order to enjoy one substantial meal.'

Dan Smith, aged 40, Worcestershire
Lost 2st 8lb (17.7kg) in 1 year and 9 months

'In November 2012, I was two months from my 40th birthday and 12st 9lb (the heaviest I've ever been) and felt that, if I was going to effect a positive change in my life, it was now or never.

'I was inspired to try the Fast Diet by two friends who achieved amazing results following the BBC programme in 2012. I needed to do something to lose weight, look and feel better. The Fast Diet made sense and appeared sustainable as a way of life rather than a short-term fix.

'The Fast Days were challenging at first, until I realised that coping with hunger is actually quite easy. I changed my relationship with food, my awareness of my diet and body, giving me control over my weight. By July 2013, I was 10st 9lb, the only downside being the need for new, smaller clothes! I have far more energy than before, have had no colds or illness and have inspired at least three others to begin their own Fast Diets.

'I feel great and genuinely in the best shape I've ever been. Thank you, Michael Mosley et al – you have changed a lot of lives for the better.'

Eleri Roberts, aged 25, Cumbria
Lost 1st (6.3kg) in 6 months

'I started the Fast Diet after watching the documentary and then reading the book. It sounded like just what I needed. I wasn't hugely overweight, I just had a few extra pounds I wanted to lose to get back into shape. Other diets put me off; the thought of giving up on treats indefinitely sounded depressing and unrealistic, so I gave 5:2 a try.

'The first few Fast Days were hard, I thought about food *all* day and fantasised about my next non-Fast Day. However, at the end of just one week I felt amazing, energised, clean and healthy.

'I soon got into a routine of saving all 500 cals for a satisfying evening meal and began to really look forward to the clean and healthy feeling gained from a Fast Day.

'In just a couple of weeks I noticed I was actually unable to eat three full meals on my five diet-free days and no longer craved so many naughty treats. Overall, in six months I have lost over a stone and reached my target weight easily. Amazing considering I have drunk wine, eaten plenty of chocolate and takeaways and had big breakfasts!

'I would recommend the 5:2 to anyone; it is not just a diet but a realistic and manageable lifestyle change.'

Britt Warg, aged 58, Swindon
Lost 1st 1lb (7kg), and has been stable for 2 years

'I started the Fast Diet just a few days after Michael Mosley's first BBC broadcast and have been sticking to it ever since, apart from a few "breaks". I have fasted two days a week – and sometimes three.

'The diet makes me feel good, happier with myself and more energetic. I have never found it hard to keep it up but at certain times, "life" has got in the way. One such period was when my mum back in Sweden was dying from Alzheimer's and I travelled back and forth over several months. I also find it difficult to turn down friends' dinner requests, especially if I am the only one invited and they have made an effort to cook.

'Before going on a sun-and-sea holiday in May this year, I made an extra effort to lose weight and managed to lose just over a stone in about three months. This was achieved by sticking to the same diet but also greatly increasing the number of regular walks I was taking. I work from home and my daily routine involves a lot of writing. I also stand up whilst working a lot more and sometimes do "silly" leg and arm movements – when nobody is watching! In shops, I take the stairs instead of escalators. I walk to the shops, instead of driving or taking the bus. Every little helps!

'Another observation: I now need less of my thyroxine tablets. I used to take 150mg but this was reduced to 125mg a year ago and more recently has been further reduced to 100mg. High cholesterol sadly runs in my family, but my levels have gone down. Also, I do a voluntary, yearly "life screening", to check for carotid artery disease, atrial fibrillation, abdominal aortic aneurysm and peripheral arterial disease. Two years ago, there was a mild plaque build up in my right carotid artery, but this year, it was back to normal.'

@iamdougroper
Thrilled to have lost a stone following @TheFastDietBook & finding 5:2 combined with exercise is good for general physical/mental health! :)

@LovellLowdown
Vastly improved my pollen allergies. Used to suffer horribly #thefastdiet

@Roband68
2 weeks into the fast diet and 2cm off the waistline and 3kg lost!!!

@mahgnilloc
16 months on fast diet and off asthma meds for the last 4 months #thefastdiet #notjustadiet

@therealjuicybug
Been a 5:2 fan for 14months & been off medication for gastric reflux problems for 12 months now. #eatclean #fastdiet

@theothersilvia
I used to be your biggest fan, but with your diet and recipes I lost 18kg, so I guess I'm a small one now.

@tracygreen72
Lost 6lb in total up to now on @TheFastDietBook (in 3 weeks and 2 days). Why didn't I discover this diet yrs ago! @DrMichaelMosley #legend

@ds14
Started in November 12, went from 12st9 to current weight of 10st1. Fitter, faster and happier than I was at 17. Now 40!

@Suethebold
@TheFastDietBook @mimispencer1 regained my confidence #nothingelseworked

@alert_bri
After 4 months on 5:2, agree with your doc assessment... this could change the world. Your book should fuel the revolution.

KEY FAST DAY INGREDIENTS

	Weight grams	Quantity/ tbsp/tsp	Total calories
PROTEIN			
Almonds		6	80
Bacon, lean	30g	1 slice	70
Chicken breast, fat removed	120g	1 medium	175
Chicken thigh, fat removed	90g	1 medium	170
Egg		1 large	90
Egg		1 medium	78
Ham, lean	45g	1 slice	60
Mackerel, fresh	150g	1 fillet	320
Mackerel, smoked	100g		202
Prawns, peeled	40g		42
Roast beef, fat removed	35g	1 slice	51
Salmon, fresh	130g	1 fillet	220
Salmon, smoked	50g		95
Sirloin steak, fat removed	140g	1 small	188
Tofu	150g		96
Trout, smoked	50g	1 fillet	75
Tuna, tinned in oil	80g		101
Tuna, tinned in spring water	80g		76
Tuna, fresh	100g	1 fillet	140
Turkey breast, cooked	35g	1 slice	39
White fish, eg cod	180g	1 fillet	175
DAIRY			
Cheddar cheese, low-fat	50g		165
Cottage cheese, low-fat	20g	1 tbsp	20

	Weight grams	Quantity/ tbsp/tsp	Total calories
Cream cheese, low-fat	35g	1 tbsp	55
Crème fraîche, low-fat	20g	1 tbsp	50g
Edam	50g		160
Feta	50g		85
Goat cheese (log)	50g		160
Milk, skimmed		1 tbsp	5
Milk, semi-skimmed	.	1 tbsp	7
Milk, almond (unsweetened)		1 tbsp	2
Milk, rice		1 tbsp	8
Milk, soy (unsweetened)		1 tbsp	5
Mozzarella, low-fat	50g		82
Parmesan, grated	10g	1 tbsp	45
Yogurt, low-fat natural yoghurt	20g	1 tbsp	15
CARBS			
Basmati rice, brown, cooked (60g uncooked)	150g		189
Basmati rice, white, cooked (60g un cooked)	130g		138
Bran flakes	40g		144
Bread, white		1 slice	96
Bread, whole-wheat		1 slice	88
Bulgur, cooked (50g dry weight)	150g		165
Couscous, cooked	100g		152
Egg noodles, cooked	150g		198
Muesli, fruit and nut	50g		177
Noodles, rice, cooked	150g		222
Noodles, shirataki	200g		4
Oats, rolled	40g		155
Potato, cooked or baked	250g	1 medium	233
Potatoes, new, boiled or steamed	200g		150
Quinoa, cooked (50g dry weight)	110g		132
Spaghetti, cooked (100g uncooked)	235g		370
Spaghetti, whole-wheat, cooked (100g uncooked)	250g		310
Tortilla, white	55g	1 tortilla	150

	Weight grams	Quantity/ tbsp/tsp	Total calories
Tortilla, wholemeal	55g	1 tortilla	144
FATS/VINEGAR			
Balsamic vinegar		1 tsp	5
Butter	7g	1 tsp	52
Olive oil		1 tsp	40
Vegetable oil		1 tsp	40
VEGGIES			
Asparagus	125g		33
Aubergine	120g		25
Avocado		½ medium	120
Baby corn	90g		22
Baked beans, low-salt and sugar	205g	½ tin	145
Bell pepper, red	160g	1 medium	50
Broccoli	100g		34
Butterbeans, cooked	120g		126
Cabbage	150g		40
Carrot	120g	1 medium	45
Cauliflower	150g		37
Celery	50g	1 stalk	8
Celeriac	250	¼ bulb	84
Cherry tomatoes	115g	10	20
Chickpeas, cooked	120g	½ tin	132
Corn on the cob	125g	1 ear	150
Courgette	150g	1 medium	33
Cucumber	100g	¼ medium	17
Fennel bulb	200g		62
French green beans	50g		16
Garlic		1 clove	3
Kidney beans, cooked	120g	½ tin	180
Leek	100g	1 large	15
Lettuce	110g		19
Mange touts	100g		18
Mushrooms, button	75g		17
Mushroom, portobello	80g	1 medium	15

	Weight grams	Quantity/ tbsp/tsp	Total calories
Olives, black or green	12g	5 medium	40
Onion	150g	1 medium	55
Peas, frozen	80g		52
Puy lentils,cooked	100g	½ tin	86
Rocket	50g		20
Spinach, fresh	100g		23
Sugar snap peas	50g		43
Sweetcorn, frozen	80g		78
Tomatoes, fresh	200g	2 medium	36
Tomatoes, tinned	200g	½ tin	44
Watercress	55g		12
FRUIT			
Apple	100g	1 small	50
Apricots	100g	2 medium	35
Apricots, dried	30gl	5 small	72
Banana	120g	1 medium	110
Blueberries	50g	20	35
Cherries	100g	10	49
Dates	25g	3 pitted	70
Fig	50g	1 medium	24
Fruit compote	100g		65-80
Grapefruit	140g	½ medium	52
Grapes	65g	10	43
Lemon juice		½ lemon	6
Lime juice		½ lime	2
Kiwi fruit	80g	1 medium	44
Melon: cantaloupe/honeydew	220g		53
Orange	160g	1 medium	70
Pear	180g	1 medium	94
Plum	55g	1 medium	24
Raisins	15g		44
Raspberries	100g	25	22
Strawberries	100g	8	30
Tangerine	80g	1 medium	25
Watermelon	300g		100

Endnotes & Research Papers

1. Longo, Valter D and Mattson, Mark. 'Fasting: Molecular mechanisms and clinical applications'. *Cell Metabolism*, 19(2), February 2014

2. Popkin, BM and Duffey, KJ. 'Does hunger and satiety drive eating anymore? Increasing eating occasions and decreasing time between eating occasions in the United States'. *American Journal of Clinical Nutrition*, May 2010

3. Kahleova, Hana. 'Eating two larger meals a day (breakfast and lunch) is more effective than six smaller meals in a reduced-energy regimen for patients with type 2 diabetes: a randomised crossover study'. *Diabetologia,* 57(8), May 2014.

4. Mattson, Mark and Calabrese, E. 'When a little poison is good for you'. *New Scientist*, August 2008

5. Carlson, AJ and Hoelzel, F, Department of Physiology, University of Chicago, US. 'Apparent prolongation of the life span of rats by intermittent fasting'. *Journal of Nutrition*, 1945.

6. Fontana, Luigi, et al, 'Medical Research: Treat Ageing'. *Nature,* July 2014

7. Bergamini, E, Cavallini, G, Donati, A and Gori, Z, Pisa, Italy. 'The role of autophagy in aging: its essential part in the anti-aging mechanism of caloric restriction'. *Annals of the New York Academy of Science,* October 2007

8. Longo, Valter D et al. 'Prolonged fasting reduces IGF-1/PKA to promote hematopoietic-stem-cell-based regeneration and reverse immunosuppression'. *Cell Stem Cell*, 14(6), June 2014

9. Varady, KA, Surabhi Bhutani, Church EC and Kempel M. 'Short-term modified alternate-day fasting: a novel dietary strategy for weight loss and cardio-protection in obese adults'. *American Journal of Clinical Nutrition*, November 2009

10. Harvie, MN, 'The effect of intermittent energy and carbohydrate restriction v. daily energy restriction on weight loss and metabolic

disease risk markers in overweight women.' *British Journal of Nutrition,* 110(8), October 2013.

11. Hussin, NM, Shahar S, Teng NIMF, Ngah WZW and Das SK. 'Efficacy of fasting and calorie restriction (FCR) on mood and depression among ageing men'. *The Journal of Nutrition, Health & Aging,* 17(8), October 2013.

12. Hatori, M, Vollmers, C, Zarrinpar, A, DiTacchio, L et al. 'Time-restricted feeding without reducing caloric intake prevents metabolic diseases in mice fed a high-fat diet'. *Cell Metabolism,* 2012

13. Erickson, KI, Voss, MW, et al, Salk Institute, San Diego, CA, US. 'Exercise training increases size of hippocampus and improves memory'. *Proceedings of the National Academy of Science USA,* January 2011

14. Halagappa, VK, Guo, Z, Pearson, M, Matsuoka, Y, Cutler, RG, Laferla, FM and Mattson, MP, National Institute on Ageing, Baltimore, MD, US. 'Intermittent fasting and caloric restriction ameliorate age-related behavioral deficits in the triple-transgenic mouse model of Alzheimer's disease'. *Neurobiology of Disease,* April 2007

15. Shirayama, Y, Chen, AC, Nakagawa, S, Russell, DS and Duman, RS, Yale University School of Medicine, New Haven, Connecticut, US. 'Brain-derived neurotrophic factor produces antidepressant effects in behavioral models of depression'. *Journal of Neuroscience,* April 2002

16. Suemaru, K, Kitamura, Y, Cui, R, Gomita, Y and Araki, H, Department of Clinical Pharmacology and Pharmacy, Brain Science, Ehime University Hospital, Japan. 'Strategy to develop a new drug for treatment-resistant depression--role of electroconvulsive stimuli and BDNF'. *Yakugaku Zasshi,* April 2007

17. Halberg, Henriksen, M, Söderhamn, N, Stallknecht, B, Ploug, T, Schjerling, P, and Dela, F, Department of Muscle Research Centre, The Panum Institute, University of Copenhagen, Denmark. 'Effect of intermittent fasting and refeeding on insulin action in healthy men'. *Journal of Applied Physiology,* December 2005

18. Raffaghello, L, Lee, C, Safdie, FM, Wei, M, Madia, F, Bianchi, G and Longo, VD, Andrus Gerontology Center, Department of Biological Sciences and Norris Cancer Center, University of Southern California, LA, CA, US. 'Starvation-dependent differential stress resistance protects normal but not cancer cells against high-dose chemo-therapy'. *Proceedings of the National Academy of Sciences of the United States of America,* June 2008

19. Lee, C, Longo, V et al, University of Southern California. 'Fasting cycles retard growth of tumours and sensitize a range of cancer cell types to chemotherapy'. *Science Translational Medicine*, February 2012

20. Safdie, F, Dorff, T, Longo, V et al, University of Southern California. 'Fasting and Cancer Treatment in Humans, *Aging,* 2009

21. Johnson, JB, Summer, W, et al. 'Alternate day calorie restriction improves clinical findings and reduces markers of oxidative stress and inflammation in overweight adults with moderate asthma'. *Free Radical Biology & Medicine*, 42(5), March 2007

22. Wolters, M. 'Diet and psoriasis: experimental data and clinical evidence'.*British Journal of Dermatology*, 153(4), Oct 2005

23. Stradling, JR, and Crosby, JH. Osler Chest Unit, Churchill Hospital, Oxford. 'Predictors and prevalence of obstructive sleep apnoea and snoring in 1001 middle-aged men'. *Thorax*, February 1991

24. Varady, KA, Bhutani, S, Klempel, MC et al. 'Alternate day fasting and endurance exercise combine to reduce body weight and favorably alter plasma lipids in obese humans'. *Obesity* (Silver Spring), 21(7), July 2013

25. Babraj, JA, Vollaard, N, Keast, C et al. 'Extremely short duration high-intensity training substantially improves the physical function and self-reported health status of an elderly population'. *Journal of the American Geriatrics Society* , 62(7), July 2014

26. Harvie, Michelle N et al, Genesis Prevention Centre, University Hospital of South Manchester NHS Foundation Trust, UK. 'The effects of intermittent or continuous energy restriction on weight loss and metabolic disease risk markers: a randomised trial in young overweight women'. *International Journal of Obesity* (London), May 2011

27. Leidy, HJ, Tang, M, Armstrong, C, Martin, CB and Campbell, WW University of Missouri, US. 'The effects of consuming frequent, higher protein meals on appetite and satiety during weight loss in overweight/obese men.' *Obesity,* 2011
&
Astrup, A, Department of Human Nutrition, Centre for Advanced Food Studies, Royal Veterinary & Agricultural University, Copenhagen, Denmark. 'The satiating power of protein – a key to obesity prevention?' *American Society for Clinical Nutrition*, July 2005
&
Halton, T and Hu, F, Department of Nutrition, Harvard School of

Public Health, Boston MA, US. 'The effects of high protein diets on thermogenesis, satiety and weight loss'. *Journal of the American College of Nutrition*, October 2004

28. Longo, V et al, 'Low protein intake is associated with a major reduction in IGF-1, cancer, and overall mortality'; *Cell Metabolism*, 19(3), March 2014

29. O'Neil, C and Nicklas, T, Louisiana State University Agricultural Center, Baton Rouge, Louisiana. 'Nut consumption Is associated with decreased health risk factors for cardiovascular disease and metabolic syndrome in US adults'. *Journal of the American College of Nutrition*, December 2011

&

Ros, E, Tapsell, LC and Sabate, J, Lipid Clinic, Endocrinology and Nutrition Service, Institut d'Investigacions Biomèdiques August Pi i Sunyer, Hospital Clínic, Barcelona, Spain. 'Nuts and berries for heart health'. *Current Atherosclerosis Reports*, November 2010

30. Dhurandhar, N, Pennington Biomedical Research Center, Louisiana, US. 'Egg proteins for breakfast keeps you feeling full for longer', May 2012

31. Wansink, B. *Mindless Eating – Why We Eat More Than We Think.* Bantam-Dell, 2006

32. Mann, T, Tomiyama AJ, Westling E, Lew A, Samuels B and Chatman J, UCLA, US. 'Medicare's search for effective obesity treatments: diets are not the answer'. *American Psychologist*, April 2007

33. Wansink, B and Sobal, J. 'Mindless eating: the 200 daily food decisions we overlook.' *Environment and Behaviour*, January 2007

34. Wansink, B, Painter, JE and Lee, Y-K. 'The Office Candy Dish: proximity's influence on estimated and actual consumption'. *International Journal of Obesity*, May 2006

35. www.marksdailyapple.com/health-benefits-of-intermittentfasting/#a xzz2DQjnYyUz

36. Van Proeyen, K, Szlufcik, K, Nielens, H, Pelgrim, K, Deldicque, L, Hesselink, M, Van Veldhoven PP, Hespel, P, Research Centre for Exercise and Health, Department of Biomedical Kinesiology, Leuven, Belgium. 'Training in the fasted state improves glucose tolerance during fat-rich diet'. *Journal of Physiology*, November 2010

37. Hollis, JF et al, Kaiser Permanente's Centre for Health Research. 'Weight loss during the intensive intervention phase of the weight-loss maintenance trial'. *American Journal of Preventive Medicine*, August 2008

38. Morewedge, CK, Young ,Eun Huh and Vosgerau, J, Carnegie Mellon University, Pittsburgh, PA, US. 'Thought for food: imagined consumption reduces actual consumption'. *Science*, December 2010

39. Fishbach, A, Eyal, T and Finkelstein, SR. 'How positive and negative feedback motivate goal pursuit'. *Social and Personality Psychology Compass*, 2010

40. Zauner, C, Schneeweiss, B, Kranz, A, Madl, C, Ratheiser, K, Kramer, L, Roth, E, Schneider, B and Lenz, K, University of Vienna, Austria. 'Resting energy expenditure in short-term starvation', *American Journal of Nutrition*, June 2000

41. Huff, MW, Robarts Research Institute at the University of Western Ontario, Canada. 'Nobiletin attenuates VLDL overproduction, dyslipidemia, and atherosclerosis in mice with diet-induced insulin resistance'. *American Journal of Diabetes*, May 2011

42. Mulvihill, EE, Alister, EM, Sutherland, BG, Telford, DE, Sawyer, CG, Edwards, JY, Markle, JM, Hegele, RA, Huff, MW. Robarts Research Institute at the University of Western Ontario, Canada. 'Naringenin prevents dyslipidemia, apoB overproduction and hyperinsulinemia in LDL-receptor null mice with diet-induced insulin resistance'. *Diabetes*, 2009

43. Fujioka, K, Greenway, F, Sheard, J and Ying, Y, Scripps Clinic, La Jolla, California, US. 'The effects of grapefruit on weight and insulin resistance: relationship to the metabolic syndrome'. *Journal of Medicinal Food*, 2006

44. Schrenk, D, Geisenheim Research Center, Germany. 'Pectin, fat absorption and anti-carcinogenic effects'. *Nutrition*, April 2008

45. Venket Rao, A and Agarwal, S, Department of Nutritional Sciences, Faculty of Medicine, University of Toronto, Canada. 'Role of antioxidant lycopene in cancer and heart disease'. *Journal of the American College of Nutrition*, October 2000

46. Karppi, J, Laukkanen, JA, Sivenius, J, Ronkainen, K and Kurl, S, Department of Medicine, Institute of Public Health and Clinical Nutrition, University of Eastern Finland, Kuopio. 'Serum lycopene decreases the risk of stroke in men'. *Neurology,* October 2012

47. Moghe, S, Texas Woman's University, Denton, Texas, US. 'Blueberries may inhibit development of fat cells'. Federation of American Societies for Experimental Biology, *Science Daily*, April 2011

48. Rolls, B and Flood, J, Penn State University, US. 'Eating soup will help cut calories at meals', presented at the Experimental Biology

Conference in Washington, May 2007

49. Liu, Rui Hai, Department of Food Science, Cornell University, Ithaca, NY, US. 'Thermal processing enhances the nutritional value of tomatoes by increasing total antioxidant activity'. *Journal of Agricultural and Food Chemistry*, April 2002

50. Miglio, C, Chiavaro, E, Visconti, A and Fogliano, V, Department of Public Health, University of Parma, Italy. 'Effects of Different Cooking Methods on Nutritional and Physicochemical Characteristics of Selected Vegetables'. *Journal of Agricultural and Food Chemistry*, December 2007

51. Herman, CP and Mack, D. 'Restrained and unrestrained eating'. *Journal of Personality*, 1975

52. Dhurandhar, EJ, Dawson, J, Alcorn, A, Larsen, LH, Thomas, E, Cardel, M, Courland, A, Astrup, A, St-Onge, M-P, Hill, J, Apovian, C, Shikany, J and Allison, D. 'The effectiveness of breakfast recommendations on weight loss: a randomized controlled trial.' *American Journal of Clinical Nutrition*, June 2014

53. Swithers, Susan E and Davidson, TL, Purdue University, West Lafayette, Indiana, US.. 'Pavlovian approach to the problem of obesity'. *International Journal of Obesity*, June 2004
&
Swithers, Susan E and Davidson, TL, Purdue University, Indiana, US. 'A role for sweet taste: calorie predictive relations in energy regulation by rats'. *Behavioral Neuroscience*, Feb 2008

54. Mesas, AE, Leon-Munoz, LM, Lopez-Garcia, E, Department of Preventive Medicine and Public Health, School of Medicine, Universidad Autónoma de Madrid, Spain. 'The effect of coffee on blood pressure and cardiovascular disease in hypertensive individuals'. *American Journal of Clinical Nutrition*, 2011
&
Larsson, S and Orsini, N, National Institute of Environmental Medicine, Karolinska Institutet, Stockholm, Sweden. 'Coffee consumption and risk of stroke: a dose-response meta-analysis of prospective studies'. *American Journal of Epidemiology*, September 2011
&
Floegel, A, Pischon, T, Bergmann, MM, Teucher, B, Kaaks, R and Boeing, H, European Prospective Investigation into Cancer and Nutrition (EPIC), Germany. 'Coffee consumption and risk of chronic disease'. *American Society for Nutrition*, April 2012

55. Kirkendall, DT, Leiper, JB, Bartagi, Z, Dvorak, J and Zerguini, Y, FIFA Medical Assessment and Research Centre, Schulthess Clinic, Zurich, Switzerland. 'The influence of Ramadan on physical performance measures in young Muslim footballers'. *Journal of Sports,* December 2008

56. Van Proeyen, K et al, Research Centre for Exercise and Health, Dept of Biomedical Kinesiology, Leuven, Belgium. 'Beneficial metabolic adaptations due to endurance exercise training in the fasted state'. *Journal of Applied Physiology*, January 2011

57. Harber, MP, Konopka, AR, Jemiolo, B, Trappe, SW, Trappe, TA and Reidy, PT, Human Performance Laboratory, Ball State University, Muncie, Indiana, US. 'Muscle protein synthesis and gene expression during recovery from aerobic exercise in the fasted and fed states'. *American Journal of Physiology,* November 2010

58. Deldicque, L, De Bock, K, Maris, M, Ramaekers, M, Nielens, H, Francaux, M and Hespel, P, Department of Biomedical Kinesiology, Leuven, Belgium. 'Increased p70s6k phosphorylation during intake of a protein-carbohydrate drink following resistance exercise in the fasted state'. *European Journal of Applied Physiology,* March 2010

59. Van Proeyen, K, Szlufcik, K, Nielens, H, Pelgrim, K, Deldicque, L, Hesselink, M, Van Veldhoven, PP and Hespel, P, Research Centre for Exercise and Health, Department of Biomedical Kinesiology, Leuven, Belgium. 'Training in the fasted state improves glucose tolerance during fat-rich diet'. *Journal of Physiology,* November 2010

60. *The New York Times,* September 15, 2010 http://well.blogs. nytimes.com/2010/12/15/phys-ed-the-benefits-ofexercising-before-breakfast/?src=me&ref=general

61. Tarnopolsky, MA, McMaster University Medical Center, Hamilton, Ontario, Canada. 'Gender differences in substrate metabolism during endurance exercise'. *Canadian Journal of Applied Physiology*, 2000

62. Stannard, SR, Buckley, AJ, Edge, JA and Thompson, MW, Institute of Food Nutrition and Human Health, Massey University, New Zealand. 'Adaptations to skeletal muscle with endurance exercise training in the acutely fed versus overnight-fasted state'. *Journal of Science and Medicine in Sport*, July 2010

Acknowledgements

This book would not have been possible without the many scientists who gave so generously of their time and their research. They include Dr Luigi Fontana of Washington University School of Medicine; Professor Mark Mattson of the National Institute on Aging; Dr Krista Varady of the University of Illinois at Chicago; and Professor Valter Longo, director of the USC Longevity Institute.

A huge thanks to Aidan Laverty, editor of BBC's *Horizon*, who pointed me towards the brave new world of intermittent fasting, and to the entire production team, but especially Kate Dart and Roshan Samarasinghe. We'd also like to thank Janice Hadlow who was brave enough to first put me in front of the camera and gave me the chance to try new things.

Thank you to Nicola Jeal at The Times for her constant ingenuity and support.

Our thanks also go to Rebecca Nicolson, Aurea Carpenter and the Short Books team, for their hard work and immediate grasp of the Fast Diet's life-changing potential.

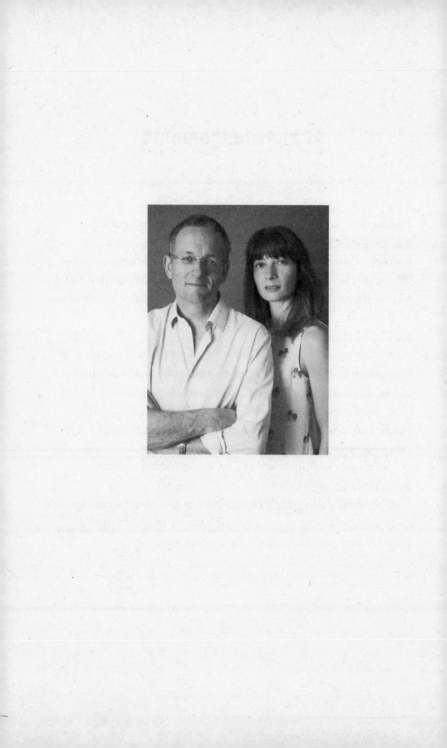

Michael Mosley did a first degree at Oxford University before training to be a doctor at the Royal Free Hospital in London. After qualifying he joined the BBC, where he has been a science journalist, executive producer and, more recently, a well-known television presenter. Unusually, he has written and presented series on BBC One, Two, Three and Four as well as BBC Radio Four. He has won numerous television awards, including an RTS, and was named Medical Journalist of the Year by the British Medical Association. He is married to a doctor and has four children, amongst them a son who is at medical school.

For more than 20 years, **Mimi Spencer** has written features for national newspapers and magazines in the UK, including *The Observer*, *The Mail on Sunday* and *The Times*. As the Fashion Editor of the *London Evening Standard*, she won the British Fashion Journalist of the Year Award in 2000, and went on to edit the paper's weekly title, *ES Magazine*.

In 2009, drawing on her personal and career interest in women's attitudes to weight loss, she wrote *101 Things to do Before You Diet* (Doubleday/Rodale).

Today, she writes regularly on women's issues and lifestyle. She lives in Brighton on the south coast of England with her husband, two children, a small boat and an endlessly hungry dog.

Index

To find out more, and for the latest science updates, recipes and tools to help you through your Fast Days, go to thefastdiet.co.uk